Chronic Non-communicable Diseases in Ghana

Multidisciplinary Perspectives

Editors
Ama de-Graft Aikins
Samuel Agyei-Mensah
Charles Agyemang

Social Science Series (Vol. 1)
Regional Institute for Population Studies

University of Ghana

UNIVERSITY OF GHANA READERS

First published in Ghana 2013 for THE UNIVERSITY OF GHANA
by **Sub-Saharan Publishers**
P.O.Box 358
Legon,Accra
Ghana
Email: saharanp@africaonline.com.gh

© University of Ghana, 2013,
P.O.Box LG 25
Legon, Accra
Ghana
Tel: +233-302-500381
website:http://www.ug.edu.gh

ISBN: 978-9988-647-27-8

Editorial Board:
Prof. (Emerita) Mary Esther Kropp Dakubu
Prof. Ama de-Graft Aikins
Prof. Kwadwo Ansah Koram
Prof. C. Charles Mate-Kole

Series Editor:
Prof. Ama de-Graft Aikins

Contents

List of Tables

Foreword

The University of Ghana is celebrating sixty-five years of its founding this year. In all those years, lecturers and researchers of the university have contributed in quite significant ways to the development of thought and in the analyses of critical issues for Ghanaian and African societies. The celebration of the anniversary provides an appropriate opportunity for a reflection on the contributions that Legon academics have made to the intellectual development of Ghana and Africa. That is the aim of the Readers Project.

In the early years of the University, all the material that was used to teach students came largely from the U.K. and other parts of Europe. Most of the thinking in all disciplines was largely Eurocentric. The material that was used to teach students was mainly European, as indeed were many of the academics teaching the students. The norms and standards against which students were assessed were influenced largely by European values. The discussions that took place in seminar and lecture rooms were driven largely by what Africa could learn from Europe.

The 1960s saw a major 'revisionism' in African intellectual development as young African academics began to question received ideas against a backdrop of changing global attitudes in the wake of political independence. Much serious writing was done by African academics as their contribution to the search for new ways of organizing their societies. African intellectuals contributed to global debates in their own right and sometimes developed their own material for engaging with their students and the wider society.

Since the late 1970s universities in the region and their academics have struggled to make their voices heard in national and global debates. Against a new backdrop of economic stagnation and political disarray, many of the ideas for managing their economies and societies have come from outside. These ideas have often come with significant financial backing channeled through international organizations and governments. During the period, African governments saw themselves as having no reason to expect or ask for any intellectual contribution from their own academics. This was very much the case in Ghana.

The story is beginning to change in African universities in many countries. The University of Ghana Readers Project is an attempt to document the different ideas that have influenced various disciplines over many years, through collections of short essays. They show the work of Legon academics and their collaborators in various disciplines as they have sought to introduce their students to new ideas. Our expectation is that this will mark a new beginning of solid engagement between Legon and other academics as they document their thoughts and contributions to the continuing search for new ideas to shape our world.

We gratefully acknowledge a generous grant from the Carnegie Corporation of New York that has made the publication of this series of Readers possible

Ernest Aryeetey
Vice-Chancellor, University of Ghana.
Legon, August 2013

Preface

Chronic non-communicable diseases (NCDs) such as hypertension, stroke, diabetes and cancers, have become major causes of adult disability and death in Ghana. They constitute public health as well as developmental challenges for the country. This edited volume presents multidisciplinary research on the major NCDs affecting Ghanaian populations. We have two key aims for this volume. First, we aim to synthesise theoretically and empirically relevant research for researchers, graduate students, healthcare providers, health policymakers and lay individuals with an interest in Ghana's burden of NCDs. We highlight and discuss the medical, psychosocial, socio-economic and policy contexts of NCDs, since the rising prevalence of these conditions have grave implications for affected individuals, families, healthcare providers and the government. Secondly, we aim to identify the limitations in current research and recommend areas for future research, practice and policy.

The chapters are multidisciplinary and multi-institutional in focus. We selected a mix of existing publications and newly commissioned chapters from leading and early career NCD researchers. This mix highlights the contemporary evolution of the field and the changing profiles of researchers and theorists. Most contributors are based at the University of Ghana, Legon, and also belong to the Academic Partnership on Chronic Conditions in Africa (APCCA), a multi-country network of social and medical scientists with an active research interest in NCDs among Africans in Sub-Saharan Africa, Europe and North America (visit www.apccafrica.org). Since 2007, network members, including the current book contributors, have collaborated on either research or publication projects relating to NCDs in Ghana and sub-Saharan Africa. The network has an institutional base at the Regional Institute for Population Studies, University of Ghana, and is managed by the first and third editors.

The volume is presented in nine chapters. Chapters 1, 2, 3, 4, 5 and 6 present syntheses of research conducted on chronic conditions of public health importance. The conditions of focus are hypertension (Juliet Addo, Charles Agyemang, Liam Smeeth and colleagues in Chapter 1), stroke (Olutobi Sanuade and Charles Agyemang in Chapter 2), diabetes (Ama de-Graft Aikins, Ellis Owusu-Dabo and Charles Agyemang in Chapter 3), cancers (Deborah Atobrah in Chapter 4), asthma (Abena Amoah, Audrey Forson and Daniel Boakye in Chapter 5) and mental health and mental disorders (Ursula Read and Victor Doku in Chapter 6). Each chapter applies either a systematic review approach or a narrative review approach to tell the story of the evolution of medical, social science or multidisciplinary research on these target conditions over a number of decades and the key insights emerging from research with respect to disease epidemiology, illness experience and healthcare implications.

Chapters 7, 8 and 9 focus on the social and policy contexts of NCDs. Unhealthy diets, overweight/obesity, physical inactivity, alcohol overconsumption and tobacco use are five risk factors, which singly or in combination, lead to major NCDs like hypertension, stroke, diabetes and cancers. In Chapter 7, Raphael Baffour Awuah and Ernest Afrifa-Anane provide a synthesis of the available evidence on the modifiable risk factors of NCDs in Ghana and show how the prevalence of risk factors has increased over time due to changing individual lifestyles, as well as structural factors such as urbanization. In chapter 8 Ama de-Graft Aikins places NCD risk, morbidity and mortality in Ghana within the African context. Focusing on the socio-cultural and socio-economic contexts of chronic diseases in the African region, she highlights the complex nature of NCD risk and experiences and the need for multi-level interventions. William Bosu, in Chapter 9, provides a historical overview of how NCD policy in Ghana has developed since the early 1990s. Bosu highlights the challenges in health policy development and offers recommendations on how these challenges can be overcome through committed and productive alliances between researchers and health policymakers.

A number of key insights emerge from this volume. First, some conditions like hypertension, diabetes and cancers, have received considerably more attention than other conditions such as asthma, stroke and neuro-degenerative conditions of ageing. Yet evidence suggests that there is a growing incidence of the latter category of chronic conditions. Secondly, the chapters indicate that for each focal condition, prevalence rates have increased, the burden on health services has increased, and complications and premature deaths are common. Thirdly, chronic disease risk, morbidity and mortality are mediated by gender, ethnicity and location. Some conditions, like stroke, affect more men than women, while others, like obesity affect more women than men. Akans, Gas and Ewes appear to have a higher prevalence of NCD risk factors like obesity, compared to other ethnic groups. There is a higher prevalence of most conditions in urban areas. Most authors emphasise the urgent need for primary, secondary and tertiary interventions for the major conditions. There is a consensus that interventions have to be multi-level and address the socio-cultural, socio-economic and gendered nature of risk, morbidity and mortality.

This edited volume offers an important overview of the public health realities and challenges of NCDs. However, a number of themes have not been subjected to chapter-length treatment. These include childhood chronic diseases, chronic neurodegenerative diseases (such as dementia, Parkinson's disease and Alzheimer's disease), access to and use of medicines, and the use of complementary and alternative medicine. These omissions are largely due to limitations in available published research in the areas. Some chapters – for example Chapter 2, Chapter 4 and Chapter 8 - deal with aspects of these themes and provide references for further reading. However, there is a need for greater research on these areas in the future.

Ama de-Graft Aikins, Samuel Agyei-Mensah and Charles Agyemang.

Contributors

Juliet Addo is clinical lecturer at the Faculty of Epidemiology and Public Health, London School of Hygiene and Tropical Medicine. She is an epidemiologist with a research focus on hypertension risk, morbidity and mortality in Ghana and the UK.

Ernest Afrifa-Anane is a PhD student at the Regional Institute for Population Studies, University of Ghana. He has an MPhil in Population Studies and is embarking on a PhD that focuses on objective and subjective measures of physical activity and its relationship to cardiovascular disease risk in Ghana.

Samuel Agyei-Mensah is professor of geography and Dean of the Faculty of Social Sciences, University of Ghana. His research focuses on medical and population geography with particular reference to the health implications of the epidemiological and fertility transitions in Ghana.

Charles Agyemang is a senior researcher and principal investigator at the Amsterdam Medical Centre, University of Amsterdam. He is a public health epidemiologist and has lead research on hypertension, obesity and risk factors of chronic non-communicable diseases among Ghanaians, Ghanaian migrants in Europe and other African populations.

Abena S. Amoah is a PhD student at the University of Leiden and research fellow at the Department of Parasitology, Noguchi Memorial Institute for Medical Research, University of Ghana.

Deborah Atobrah is a research fellow at the Institute of African Studies, University of Ghana. She is an anthropologist with a major research interest in lay perceptions and management of terminal conditions.

Raphael Baffour Awuah is a PhD student at the Regional Institute for Population Studies. He has an MPhil in Population Studies and is embarking on a PhD that focuses on the gendered context and impact of cardiovascular disease in Ghana.

Daniel A. Boakye is professor of entomology and parasitology at the Noguchi Memorial Institute for Medical Research. His research interests include the control of vectorborne diseases and neglected tropical Diseases (e.g.

lymphatic filariasis, onchocerciasis) and the role of parasitic infections in the modulation of the immune response to allergic disorders.

William K. Bosu is the immediate past manager of Ghana's Non-Communicable Disease Control Programme (NCDCP). He now heads the NCD unit at the West African Health Organization (WAHO). He is an epidemiologist and public health specialist and has conducted research on hypertension and risk factors of NCDs.

Ama de-Graft Aikins is associate professor of social psychology at the Regional Institute for Population Studies and Director of the Centre for Social Policy Studies, University of Ghana. Her research interests include diabetes experiences and care, food beliefs and habits, health and illness representations and the development of community-based cardiovascular disease (CVD) interventions.

Victor Doku is a consultant psychiatrist affiliated with the Institute of Psychiatry, University of London. He has conducted research on severe mental illness and epilepsy and facilitated capacity development programmes on mental health training in Ghana.

Anthony K. Edusei is a senior lecturer at the School of Medical Sciences, Kwame Nkrumah University of Science and Technology.

Audrey Forson is a pulmonary physician based at the Department of Medicine, University of Ghana Medical School. Her research interests include asthma and related chronic respiratory conditions.

Gbenga Ogedegbe is professor and Director of the Center for Healthful Behaviour Change at New York University. He is a public health specialist with a research interest in hypertension among African, African-American and Caribbean communities in the US and among Ghanaians in Ghana.

Ellis Owusu-Dabo is senior lecturer at the School of Medical Sciences and Scientific Director of the Kumasi Collaborative Centre for Research on Tropical Diseases (KCCR), Kwame Nkrumah University of Science and Technology. He is a medical scientist and public health specialist with a research interest in the interface between infectious diseases and chronic non-communicable diseases.

Ursula M. Read is a career development fellow at the Medical Research Council, University of Glasgow. She is an anthropologist with a research focus on experiences of severe mental illness in Ghana and the UK.

Oluwatobi Sanuade is a PhD student at the Regional Institute for Population Studies. He has an MPhil in Population Studies and is embarking on a PhD that focuses on the burden and psychosocial impact of stroke in Ghana.

Liam Smeeth is professor of clinical epidemiology and head of the Department of Non-communicable Disease Epidemiology, London School of Hygiene and Tropical Medicine. His research interests include non-communicable disease epidemiology in low-income countries, with a particular focus on cardiovascular disease.

Abbreviations

APCCA	Academic Partnership on Chronic Conditions in Africa
APH	Accra Psychiatric Hospital
CMDs	Common mental disorders
CNCDs	Chronic non-communicable diseases
CSRPM	Centre for Scientific Research into Plant Medicine
DHIMS	District Health Information Management Systems
DSM	Diagnostic and Statistical Manual of Mental Disorders
ECOWAS	Economic Community of West African States
FCTC	Framework Convention on Tobacco Control
GDA	Ghana Diabetes Association
GDHS	Ghana Demographic and Health Survey
GHS	Ghana Health Service
GLSS	Ghana Living Standards Survey
GMA	Ghana Medical Association
GNA	Ghana News Agency
ICD	International Classification of Diseases
IDF	International Diabetes Federation
IDSR	Integrated Disease Surveillance and Response
ISAAC	International Study of Asthma and Allergy in Childhood
KATH	Komfo Anokye Teaching Hospital
KBTH	Korle-Bu Teaching Hospital
LMICs	Low- and Middle- Income Countries
MDGs	Millennium Development Goals
MOH	Ministry of Health
NCD	Non-communicable Disease
NCDCP	Non-communicable Disease Control Programme
NHIA	National Health Insurance Authority
NHIS	National Health Insurance Scheme
RHNP	Regenerative Health and Nutrition Programme
RODAM	Risk of Obesity and Diabetes among African Migrants
SAGE	Study on Global Ageing and Adult Health
SSA	Sub-Saharan Africa
WHA	World Health Assembly
WHO	World Health Organization
WHO-Afro	World Health Organization, Africa Region
WHO AUDIT	WHO Alcohol Use Disorders Identification Test
WHO-PEN	WHO Package of Essential NCD Interventions
WHS	World Health Survey

MAP OF GHANA SHOWING HEALTH SERVICES

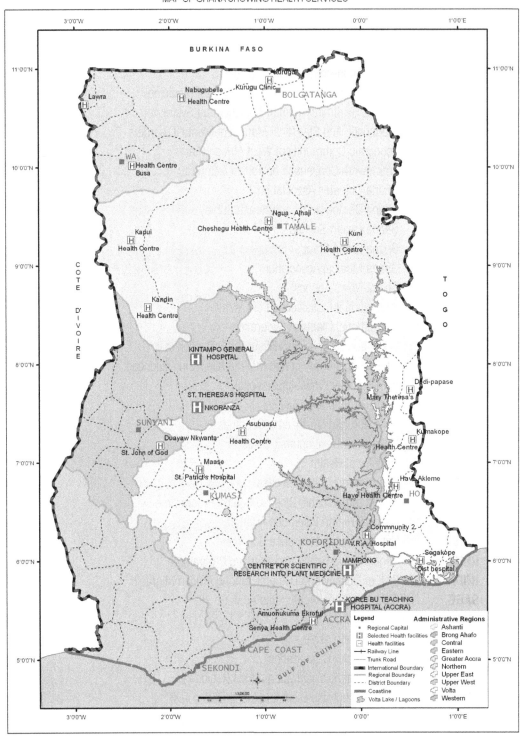

Introduction:

Multidisciplinary perspectives on chronic non-communicable diseases in Ghana

Ama de-Graft Aikins, Samuel Agyei-Mensah and Charles Agyemang

There is a general notion among Ghanaian experts and lay communities that the major public health problems affecting Ghanaians are infectious diseases, malnutrition and maternal and child mortality. The reality is much more complex. In the late 19th century, European anthropologists recorded sickle cell-disease and asthma in Asante communities (Addae, 1996), but prior to this, lay communities recognized and named both conditions (Konotey-Ahulu, 1991). In the 1920s hypertension cases were presented to the newly built Korle Bu hospital (Pobee, 2004), even as infectious diseases like malaria and tuberculosis caused immense suffering among the indigenous Ga communities of Accra (Patterson, 1979). In the 1950s, while Western psychiatrists proposed theories about the lack of mental illness in African societies, a range of acute and chronic mental health disorders were recognized, named and treated by families and traditional healers (de-Graft Aikins, 2013; Field, 1960; Jahoda, 1961; Read et al., 2013). Since these early colonial records, Ghana's public health profile has been characterized by a co-existence of infectious and chronic diseases. Hospital-based medical research in Accra and Kumasi in the 1950s and 1960s recorded cases of hypertension, stroke, cancers and sickle-cell disease alongside malaria, diarrhoea and other infectious diseases (Agyei-Mensah and de-Graft Aikins, 2010; de-Graft Aikins, 2007). Community-based studies during the same period in the Brong-Ahafo Region recorded cases of mild and severe mental health disorders (Field, 1960). Over subsequent decades, the hospital-based data have shown a systematic increase in out-patient and mortality rates due to hypertension, stroke and diabetes. When community-based research was introduced in the 1960s in Accra, Ho and Kumasi, the prevalence of conditions like diabetes and hypertension was low, but these rates have also increased significantly, like that recorded for hospitals (see Addo et al. in Chapter 2; de-Graft Aikins et al., Chapter 3; Bosu, Chapter 9). Hypertension prevalence is now estimated at 37 percent in urban areas and 24 percent in rural areas (see

Addo et al., Chapter 2). Diabetes prevalence rates range between 6 percent and 8 percent and peaks at around 9.1 percent among urban civil servants (see de-Graft Aikins et al., Chapter 3). The prevalence of common mental disorders (mainly depression and anxiety disorders) is estimated at 10 percent, while severe mental disorders (psychosis, schizophrenia) is estimated at 3 percent. In sharp contrast to these NCD prevalence rates, HIV prevalence is less than 2 percent currently. However, HIV/AIDS and other infectious diseases are prioritized for ring-fenced funding and health-system interventions, while NCDs are neglected.

Ghana's chronic disease burden has complex, multifaceted roots and consequences. Urbanisation, rapidly ageing populations, globalisation, poverty, poor lifestyle practices and weak health systems have been identified as key intersecting factors. The development of research, intervention and policy solutions has to be informed by the complexity of the problem. In this introductory chapter, we make a case for the importance of developing a multidisciplinary approach to NCD research and intervention in Ghana. The chapter is presented in two parts. The global burden of NCDs, particularly in low- and middle-income countries (LMICs), has been attributed to a health transition made up of interlinked demographic, epidemiological and nutrition transitions. Ghana, like many LMICs, is experiencing a health transition. Its NCD burden must, therefore, be understood within this context. In the first part of the chapter we present available evidence that links the rising NCD burden to demographic, epidemiological and nutritional changes at population level. The relationship between factors such as a growing ageing population (demographic transition), diseases linked to urban poverty (epidemiological transition) and the impact of food market globalization on nutritional status and body weight (nutrition transition) suggests that multidisciplinary research is needed to understand NCD risk, experience and interventions. In the second part of the chapter, we provide a brief history of NCD research and highlight the evolution of research from a field dominated by medical science to one opening up to multidisciplinary collaborative projects. We review the extent to which the available research has addressed NCD risk, morbidity and mortality and we outline future prospects and challenges in the field.

The health transition and NCDs in Ghana

The coexistence of infectious diseases and chronic diseases in Ghana has been attributed to a health transition that is common to many LMICs (Agyei-Mensah and de-Graft Aikins, 2010; Frenk et al., 1989; Maher et al., 2010). The health transition has been attributed to a confluence of demographic, epidemiological and nutritional transitions. The complex dynamics of these transitions highlight the complex and multi-level roots and consequences of NCDs.

The demographic transition has been defined as a transition of populations that are largely rural and young with high fertility rates to populations that are ageing and urbanised with low fertility rates. Ghana's demographic profile mirrors this transition. Ghana's ageing population has trebled over the last thirty years, urban populations have increased exponentially and the country's fertility level, at 4, is one of the lowest on the continent (Ayernor, 2012; Agyei-Mensah and de-Graft Aikins, 2010; Agyei-Mensah, 2006; Mba, 2010). These demographic trends are similar to trends in other African countries. Urbanisation and ageing present major implications for the health profile of countries. Urbanisation comes with the stresses of urban living, including congested built environments (for the urban poor), sedentary work patterns, poor lifestyle practices (such as alcohol use, smoking and poor eating practices) and social isolation. Poverty, a key feature of urbanization in many African countries, including Ghana, is associated with social tensions, psychological insecurities and mental health problems (de-Graft Aikins and Ofori-Atta, 2007; Grief et al., 2011). However, there is increasing recognition that poverty is also associated with the double jeopardy of infectious and chronic disease. Since the 1970s, studies in Accra have shown that poor communities experience a dual risk of infectious and chronic diseases compared to wealthier communities that are predisposed largely to chronic diseases (Pobee, 2006; Agyei-Mensah and de-Graft Aikins, 2010). Poor communities living with chronic diseases are also likely to suffer greater complications and die prematurely because they lack access - in geographical, economic and cultural terms - to quality healthcare. Ageing increases the risk of chronic physical and neurodegenerative diseases like Parkinson's disease, Alzheimer's disease and dementia, and complex neurological conditions associated with strokes. Common problems recorded among the ageing population by the Study on Global Ageing and Adult Health (SAGE) conducted in 2005, included oral health problems, hypertension, arthritis, diabetes, hypertension and related cardiovascular conditions (Ayernor, 2012).

Co-morbidities were common. Rural-urban migration is largely a livelihood and lifestyle choice of the youth. Therefore, there are more older people living in rural areas than in urban areas. Analysis of the SAGE data showed that more rural older individuals were living with NCDs. This has implications for access to and quality of healthcare for the elderly, who are likely to live with co-morbid and multi-morbid conditions.

The epidemiological transition has been defined as the complex changes that occur with patterns of health and diseases, how these patterns interact and the underpinning demographic, economic and sociological factors and consequences (Omran, 1971). Omran (1971) proposed a classic model of epidemiological transition which suggested that countries would transition, sequentially, from periods of high death rates due to infectious diseases to high death rates due to chronic and degenerative diseases of ageing. Various permutations of Omran's model have been proposed. Among these, the Protracted Polarised Model of epidemiological transition, proposed by Frenk and colleagues (1989), is regarded as the most relevant for countries of Africa, Asia and Latin America. In this model, both infectious and chronic and degenerative diseases of ageing are major causes of morbidity and mortality. This occurs for two reasons. The "protracted" aspect of the model describes partial changes to the patterns of morbidity and mortality due to the co-existence of infectious diseases (both traditional and new) and chronic non-communicable diseases. The "polarized" aspect describes the relationship between socio-economic status and disease risk, whereby wealthy communities live with the risk of chronic diseases of lifestyle, while poor communities live with the dual risk of chronic diseases of lifestyle and infectious diseases of poverty.

Agyei-Mensah and de-Graft Aikins (2010) reviewed multidisciplinary research conducted in Accra between 1877 and the mid-2000s to examine the nature of the epidemiological transition in the capital. They reported that the transition in Accra reflected the protracted polarised model and attributed this profile to a combination of urbanization, urban poverty and globalization. The authors hypothesised that similar trends were likely to pertain to other African cities.

The nutrition transition occurs when countries and communities simultaneously experience over-nutrition (diets high in energy, saturated fat, cholesterol, and sodium, but low in fibre) and under-nutrition (diets low in either energy or various specific nutrients including niacin, riboflavin, vitamin C, zinc, calcium and magnesium) (Popkin et al., 2011; Amuna and Zotor, 2008). Over-nutrition has been attributed to food market globalization and urbanisation, both contributing to changing dietary practices and the rise in overweight and obesity. Under-nutrition is attributed predominantly to poverty, in terms of a fundamental lack of access to nutritious food. The Ghana Demographic and Health Surveys conducted between 1988 and 2008 (at five-year intervals) have recorded high levels of over-nutrition among women in urban areas of the Greater Accra, Ashanti and Western regions and under-nutrition among women and children in rural areas and the Northern, Upper East and Upper West regions (GDHS, 1988, 2003, 2008). Crucially, as the global literature suggests, over-nutrition and under-nutrition can co-exist within communities, households and individuals (Popkin et al., 2011). Poor households, for example, may have over-nourished obese adults and undernourished underweight children. Or individuals may experience both over-nutrition and under-nutrition because their diet is simultaneously high in energy and saturated fat and low in key micro-nutrients. Over-nutrition and under-nutrition both raise the risk of major chronic diseases. Over-nutrition is a major risk factor for overweight and obesity, which in turn are risk factors for major conditions like diabetes, stroke and cancers. Under-nutrition is also associated with atypical diabetes, cardiovascular diseases and some cancers. Childhood under-nutrition is reported to raise the risk of adult obesity (Amuna and Zotor, 2008).

The relationship between these transitions and common NCDs suggests that NCD risk has to be understood as a product of structural, environmental and historical processes as well as a product of individual choices and behaviour. Similarly, while NCD experiences constitute medical problems affecting individuals, their impact transcend affected individuals. Chronic illness experiences are embedded in the social world of the chronically ill. Knowledge, attitudes, motivations and actions relating to the lived condition operate within, and are mediated by, the social world. Thus, illness experiences, and individual responses to illness experiences, are better understood when research is informed by integrated medical and social science approaches.

Multidisciplinary research on NCDs in Ghana

NCD research in Ghana was dominated by medical science from the 1920s to the 1980s. During the first thirty years of the publication of the Ghana Medical Journal, between the 1960s and 1990s, specific disease areas were synonymous with specific medical scientists (de-Graft Aikins and Tagoe, 2009). For example sickle cell disease research was synonymous with Konotey-Ahulu, diabetes was synonymous with Dodu, Owusu and Amoah and hypertension with Pobee. A limited number of in-depth anthropological and social history studies on general health, mental health and social practices were conducted during this period and offered an important socio-cultural context for understanding the medical trends (cf. Akyeampong, 1996; Field, 1937, 1960; Mullings, 1984). For example Field's anthropological work on Ga communities in the 1930s outlined general health and illness beliefs that provided insights on chronic disease risk and the nature of social support for the chronically ill (Field, 1937). Similarly, Field's ethnographic work on mental health in Brong Ahafo in the 1950s provided important evidence on local constructions of depression, particularly among ageing women (Field, 1960). Mullings' 1970s study of mental health and mental healing among Ga communities highlighted the utility of traditional healing practice, including the emerging role of charismatic Christian healing repertoires. However, these studies were isolated from the medical research being conducted at the time and their insights were not incorporated into the growing concerns about chronic illness management, the use of traditional medicine and the role of social support.

A distinct social science focus on NCDs emerged in the 1990s. This focus coincided with emerging policy attention on the health systems impact of NCDs (see Bosu, Chapter 9). Since the late 1990s, the number of social science studies on NCDs has increased steadily. Doctoral and masters'-level projects have been conducted on NCDs from psychology, anthropology, public health and population studies perspectives. These projects and wider studies have focused on a growing range of socio-cultural issues relating to cancers, diabetes, hypertension and sickle-cell disease including population and community prevalence, lay knowledge, lived experiences, and the development of interventions (cf. Abanilla et al., 2010; Atobrah, 2012; Ayernor, 2012; de-Graft Aikins, 2003, 2005; Dennis-Antwi et al., 2011; Kratzer, 2012; Spencer et al., 2005; Tagoe, 2012). Empirical studies have been conducted in the Greater Accra Region (Accra, Tema), Ashanti Region (Kumasi), Brong-Ahafo Region (Kintampo, Nkoranza) and the Western Region (Takoradi). Some social science studies, including graduate projects, have been embedded in funded multidisciplinary collaborative projects. Major collaborative studies include the Accra Women's Health Study (e.g. Darko et al., 2012; Hill et al., 2007; see also Chapter 2), the New York University-Regional Institute for Population Studies (NYU-RIPS) collaborative project on cardiovascular disease task-shifting and nutrition interventions (Awuah et al, submitted; see also Chapter 3) and the Risk of Obesity and Diabetes among African Migrants (RODAM) Study (Agyemang et al, 2012; see also Chapter 3). These projects provide an important new model of NCD research in Ghana. They move research from isolated hubs of medical and social science studies to integrated projects that examine the complex roots and public health implications of NCDs. They offer the necessary multi-level evidence to aid the development of appropriate interventions.

Conclusions

NCDs constitute a major public health problem for Ghanaians. The roots of the problem do not lie solely in individual lifestyles, as is commonly reported, but also within structural and environmental systems. Ultimately, NCDs present a unique contemporary public health challenge that requires dismantling of the old standard ways of researching disease and illness experience and of providing healthcare in Ghana. These diseases should be understood from two broad, and integrated, perspectives: the medical and the social. The medical perspective focuses on the biological event of disease and its targeted treatment. The social perspective focuses on the everyday dimensions of disease risk and experiences, which encompasses the psychological, spiritual, socio-cultural and economic. For the individual living with a chronic condition, the medical and social dimensions of their condition are inextricably linked and shape everyday experiences, self-care and health outcomes. Research therefore needs to move beyond a predominantly clinical approach that prioritizes the biological basis of disease to a more multidisciplinary and multi-institutional approach to NCD research that focuses on the biological, psychological, socio-cultural and spiritual. The healthcare system needs to prioritize prevention alongside cure or therapeutic approaches. The role of complementary and alternative medical systems in NCD care needs to be properly understood and incorporated into NCD policy.

Disease is not only a matter of public health; it is also a matter of human and national development. When large numbers of children and adults get sick and die prematurely from preventable diseases, this adversely affects the structure and quality of life of families, the levels of productivity in the workplace and the development goals and processes of nations. Thus, as local experts have argued, NCDs do not only constitute a major public health problem for Ghanaians, but also constitute a developmental problem for the nation. Experts argue that without the development and implementation of the appropriate research approaches, interventions and policies, the rising burden of chronic diseases will cripple health systems, reverse the gains made on the Millennium Development Goals (MDGs) (especially MDG1, MDG5 and MDG6[1]), and create significant challenges for governance and development (Beaglehole et al. 2011).

The public health and developmental impact of NCDs has been a major topic of policy debate globally since the mid-1990s (Beaglehole et al, 2011; Fuster and Vote, 2005; Horton, 2005; Unwin et al., 2001; WHO, 2005). Two decades of research syntheses, international meetings and WHO advocacy, culminated in a high-level meeting (HLM) on NCDS convened by the United Nations in New York in September 2011. The UN HLM on NCDs focused on the developmental implications of NCDs on low- and middle -income countries of Africa, Asia and Latin America. Governments, including that of Ghana, signed up to a 'whole-of-government, whole-of-society' policy approach to tackling the rising burden of NCDs in their countries.

This approach followed a longstanding recommendation for low- and middle-income countries to develop multi-level and multi-institutional responses to their NCD crises. The multi-level aspect takes into account the individual, group, community and structural dimensions of NCD risk, morbidity and mortality. The multi-institutional aspect takes into account the synergistic relationships between various institutions involved in the everyday health of populations and the provision of healthcare and NCD care, including health centres, faith-based organizations, workplaces, the mass media, research institutions and policymaking bodies. This multi-level, multi-institutional approach to interventions is required because the financial and psychosocial costs of living with NCDs in Ghana are high and they push a growing number of affected individuals and families into poverty, social isolation and poor physical and mental health outcomes.

---

1   MDG1 (eradicate extreme poverty and hunger), MDG5 (improve maternal health), MDG6 (combat HIV/AIDS, malaria and other diseases).

References

Abanilla, P.K.A., Huang, K-Y, Shinners, S, Levy, A, Kojo Ayernor, K., de-Graft Aikins, A, Ogedegbe, O. (2011). Cardiovascular Disease Prevention in Ghana: Feasibility of a Faith-Based Organizational Approach to Prevention. *Bulletin of the World Health Organization*, 89, 648-656.

Addae, S.(1996).*History of Western Medicine in Ghana, 1880 – 1960*. Durham: Durham Academic Press.

Adubofuor, K.O.M., Ofei, F., Mensah-Adubofour, J., Owusu, S.K.. Diabetes in Ghana: a morbidity and mortality analysis. *International Diabetes Digest* 1993; 4(3), 90-92.

Adubofour KOM, Ofei, F., Mensah-Adubufour J, Owusu SK. Diabetes in Ghana. In Gill G, Mbanya J-C, Alberti G (Eds), *Diabetes in Africa*. 1997; FSG Communications Ltd, Reach, Cambridge, UK. (pp. 83-88).

Agyei-Mensah, S. and de-Graft Aikins, A. (2010). Epidemiological transition andthe double burden of disease in Accra, Ghana. *Journal of Urban Health, 87 (5), 879-897.*

Akyeampong, E.K (1996). *Drink, Power and Cultural Change: A Social History of Alcohol in Ghana, c.1800 to Recent Times*. Portsmouth: Heinemann.

Alwan, A., Maclean, D. and Mandil, A. (2001).*Assessment of National Capacity for Noncommunicable Disease Prevention and Control.* 2001. Geneva: WHO.

Amoah, A.G.B, Owusu, K.O., and Adjei, S. (2002) Diabetes in Ghana: a community prevalence study in Greater Accra. *Diabetes Research and Clinical Practice*, 2002; 56: 197-205.

Amoah, A.G.B. (2003a) Obesity in adult residents of Accra, Ghana. *Ethnicity and Disease*, 2003a; 13(2 Suppl 2): S29-101.

Amoah, A.G.B. (2003b) Sociodemographic variations in obesity among Ghanaian adults. *Public Health Nutrition*, 6(8): 751-775.

Amuna, P. And Zotor, F.B. (2008). Epidemiological and nutrition transition in developing countries: impact on human health and development. *Proceedings of the Nutrition Society*, 67, 82-90.

Atobrah, D. (2012) When darkness falls at mid-day: Young patients' perceptions and meanings of chronic illness and their implications for medical care. *Ghana Medical Journal, 46(2)*, 46-53.

Ayernor, P.K (2012). Diseases of ageing in Ghana. *Ghana Medical Journal*, 46(2), 18-22.

Beaglehole, R., Bonita, R., Horton, R., Adams, C., Alleyne, G. et al (2011). Priority actions for the non-communicable disease crisis. *Lancet*; 377: 1438–47

Biritwum, R.B., Gyapong, J. and Mensah, G. The epidemiology of obesity in Ghana. *Ghana Medical Journal*, 2005; 39, 3, 82-85.

Cappuccio FP, Micah FB, Emmett L, Kerry SM, Antwi S, Martin-Peprah R, Phillips RO, Plange-Rhule J, and Eastwood JB. (2004). Prevalence, detection, management, and control of hypertension in Ashanti, West Africa. *Hypertension*. 43(5):1017-22.

Debpuur C, Welaga P, Wak G, Hodgson A. (2010). Self-reported health and functional limitations among older people in the Kassena-Nankana District, Ghana. *Global Health Action*, 27(3).

Dennis-Antwi, J.A., Culley, L., Hiles, D.R and Dyson, S.M. (2011). 'I can die today, I can die tomorrow': lay perceptions of sickle cell disease in Kuamsi, Ghana at a point of transition. *Ethnicity and Health*, 16(4-5), 465-81. de-Graft Aikins, A. (2005). Healer-shopping in Africa: new evidence from a rural-urban qualitative study of Ghanaian diabetes experiences. *British Medical Journal*, 331, 737.

de-Graft Aikins, A and Tagoe, H. (2009). *Bibliography on non-communicable diseases research in Ghana: 1950-2009*. Available at www.appcafrica.org.

de-Graft Aikins, A., Unwin, N., Agyemang, C. Allotey, P., Campbell, C and Arhinful, D.K. (2010). Tackling Africa's Chronic Disease Burden: from the local to the global. *Globalization and Health*, 6:5.

de-Graft AikinsA., Arhinful, D.K., Pitchforth, E., Ogedegbe, O., Allotey, P., Agyemang, C. (2012). Establishing and Sustaining Research Partnerships in Africa: a case study of the UK-Africa Academic Partnership on Chronic Disease. *Globalization and Health*, 8: 29.

Dodu, S.R.A and de Heer, N. (1964).A diabetes case-finding survey in Ho. *Ghana Medical Journal*, 1964; 3:75-80.

Ferri, C., Chisholm, D., Van Ommeren, M., Prince, M. (2004).Resource utilisation for neuropsychiatric disorders in developing countries: a multinational Delphi consensus study. *Soc Psychiatry Psychiatr Epidemiol*.39(3):218-27.

Frenk J, Bobadilla, J.L, Sepulveda, J., Cervantes, M.L. (1989). Health transition in middle-income countries: new challenges for health care. *Health Policy Plan*. 4(1): 29-39.

Fuster, V and Voûte. (2005). MDGs: chronic diseases are not on the agenda. *Lancet*, 366.

Ghana Statistical Service (GSS), Noguchi Memorial Institute for Medical Research (NMIMR), and ORC Macro (2004). *Ghana Demographic and Health Survey 2003*. Calverton, Maryland: GSS, NMIMR, and ORC Macro.

Horton, R. (2005).The neglected epidemic of chronic disease. *Lancet*, 366.

Jahoda, G. (1961). Traditional healers and other institutions concerned with mental health in Ghana. *International Journal of Social Psychiatry*, 7: 245-268.

Kowal, P., Kahn, K., Ng, N., Naidoo, N., Abdullah, S. et al. (2010). Ageing and adult health status in eight lower-income countries: the INDEPTH WHO-SAGE collaboration. *Global Health Action*, 27;3.

Maher, D, Smeeth, L, Sekajugo, J. (2010). Health transition in Africa: practical policy proposals for primary care. *Bulletin of the World Health Organization*, 88: 943-948

Mba, C.J. (2010). Population ageing in Ghana: research gaps and the way forward. *Journal of Ageing Research*, 29.

Ministry of Health (MOH) (Ghana). *The health of the nation. Analysis of Health sector programme of work: 1997-2001. 2001*. Accra: MOH.

MOH (Ghana) (2005). *Creating Wealth Through Health*. Minister's Press Briefing, Accra: MOH.

MOH (Ghana) (2007). *The Ghana Health Sector 2007 Programme of Work*. Accra: MOH.

Moussavi, S., Chatterji,S., Verdes,E., Tandon, A., Patel, V., and Ustun, B.(2007). Depression, chronic diseases, and decrements in health:results from the World Health Surveys. *Lancet*; 370: 851–58

Mullings, L. (1984). Therapy, Ideology and Social Change: Mental Healing in Urban Ghana. Berkeley: University of California Press

Omran A.R.(1971).The epidemiological transition theory: a theory of the epidemiology of population change. *Milbank Mem Fund Q.* 49: 6-47.

Pobee, J.O.M. (2006).*The Heart of the Matter. Community Profile of Cardiovascular Diseases of a sub-Saharan African Country*. Accra: Commercial Associates Ltd.

Popkin, B.M, Adair, L.S, and Ng SW. (2012). Global nutrition transition and the pandemic of obesity in developing countries. *Nutritional Reviews*; 70(1):3-21.

Setel, P.W. (2003). Non-communicable diseases, political economy, and culture in Africa: anthropological applications in an emerging pandemic. *Ethnicity and Disease*,13(2 Suppl 2):S149-57.

Spencer J, Phillips E, Ogedegbe G. (2005). Knowledge, attitudes, beliefs, and blood pressure control in a community-based sample in Ghana. *Ethnicty and Disease*, 15:748-52.

Strong, K., Mathers, C., Leeder, S. and Beaglehole, R..(2005). Preventing chronic diseases: how many lives can we save? *Lancet* .published online Oct 5.DOI:10.1016/S0140 6736(05)67341-2

Tagoe, H.A. (2012). Household burden of chronic diseases in Ghana. *Ghana Medical Journal*, 46(2), 54-58.

Turkson, S.N., and Asamoah, V. (1997).Common psychiatric disorders among the elderly attending a general psychiatric out patient clinic in Accra, Ghana: a five year retrospective study (1989-1993).*West Africa Journal of Medicine*, 16(3), 146-9.

Unwin, N., Setel, P., Rashid, S., Mugusi, F., Mbanya, J., Kitange, H., Hayes, L., Edwards, R., Aspray, T. and Alberti, K.G.M.M. (2001). Noncommunicable diseases in sub-Saharan Africa: where do they feature in the health research agenda? *Bulletin of the World Health Organisation*. 79(10), 947-953.

Unwin, N. and Alberti, K.G.M.M. (2006). Chronic non-communicable diseases. *Annals of Tropical Medicine and Pharmacology.* 100 (5 & 6), 455-464.

World Health Organization (WHO) (2005).*Preventing Chronic Disease.A vital investment.*Geneva: WHO.

WHO/FAO (2003). Diet, nutrition and the prevention of chronic diseases: report of a joint WHO/FAO expert Consultation. Geneva: WHO.

Chapter 1

A review of population-based studies on hypertension in Ghana[1]

Juliet Addo, Charles Agyemang, Liam Smeeth, Ama de-Graft Aikins, A. K. Edusei and Gbenga Ogedegbe

Introduction

Hypertension is an important public health challenge in both economically developing and developed countries (Kearney et al., 2004). It is becoming an increasingly common health problem because of increasing longevity and prevalence of contributing factors such as obesity, physical inactivity and an unhealthy diet (Ezzati et al., 2005; Singh et al., 2000; Yusuf et al., 2001). The current prevalence of hypertension in many developing countries, particularly in urban societies, is reported to be already as high as is seen in developed countries (Khor, 2001; Vorster, 2002; Addo et al., 2007). The prevalence of hypertension is expected to increase even further in the absence of broad and effective preventive measures (Chobanian et al., 2003).

This is especially true for Ghana where hypertension was reported to be the second leading cause of outpatient morbidity in adults older than 45 years in Ghana (MOH, 2005). At the leading teaching hospital in Ghana between 1990 and 1997, non-communicable diseases and their complications accounted for more than two-thirds of all medical admissions and more than 50 percent of all deaths (MOH, 2005). An increase in morbidity associated with hypertension not only reflects a high prevalence of hypertension, but is also an indication of inadequate rates of detection, treatment and control. In an examination of post-mortem records in the Korle Bu Teaching Hospital in Accra between 1994 and 1998, 11 percent of deaths in adults aged 20 years or more were due to stroke, most of which were haemorrhagic (Wiredu and Nyame, 2001). Hypertension was a predominant factor in these strokes.

---

1   Previously published as Addo, J., Agyemang, C., Smeeth, L., de-Graft Aikins, A., Edusei, A.K., Ogedegbe, O. (2012). A review of population-based studies on hypertension in Ghana. *Ghana Medical Journal,* 46 (2), 4-11.

Most of the hypertension research to date has been undertaken among white participants in developed country settings. Health service factors relating to the detection and control of hypertension and environmental determinants of blood pressure such as diet and physical activity - differ markedly between Africa and most Western settings. In addition, there is some evidence that compared to white people, people of black African origin have higher risk of developing hypertension, the blood pressure elevation is often more marked and more rapid and that achieving blood pressure control is more difficult (Brown, 2006). Reliable information about the prevalence of hypertension in different world regions is essential to the development of health policies for prevention and control of this condition (Kearney et al., 2005). The absence of reliable data on the prevalence of major cardiovascular risk factors in

(SSA), let alone the trends over time, has been identified as a major impediment to developing appropriate policies and interventions to prevent and treat cardiovascular disease (CVD) in the region (Beaglehole, 2001; Unwin et al., 2001; Yach et al., 2005; Mendis et al., 2003; Bonita and Douglas, 2001). Current estimates and projections around non-communicable diseases for most of SSA are largely based on assumptions and extrapolations (Mathers and Loncar, 2006; Rodgers et al., 2004).

The purpose of this review was to identify population-based studies of hypertension in Ghana; to determine the prevalence, detection, treatment and control rates reported in these studies; examine the sex and urban-rural differences, if any, in these rates; examine temporal trends in the prevalence, detection, treatment and control of hypertension and to examine the factors associated with hypertension and its control.

Methods

A literature search of the PUBMED database was conducted from 1970 to 2009 using the medical subject headings "hypertension", blood pressure" and "Ghana". A manual search for additional studies was performed using references cited in the original articles. Additionally, we contacted some key researchers working on hypertension in Ghana for studies known to them which might have been missed. The review was limited to population-based studies involving Ghanaians aged 15 years and above. Data were extracted following a standard protocol and using standard data collection forms and a checklist by a single reviewer. Variables extracted included year of survey, age of participants, sampling methods, response rate, sample size, methods for preparation and measurement of blood pressure, definition(s) used for hypertension, and type of measuring device used. The mean systolic (SBP) and diastolic blood pressure (DBP), prevalence of hypertension (unadjusted and age adjusted), percentage of participants with previously diagnosed hypertension, those on treatment and those whose blood pressure was controlled (BP<140/90 mmHg) were also obtained. Where information was available we described the population used for the standardization of hypertension prevalence, and categorized the prevalence of hypertension by gender and rural-urban residence. Multiple papers from a study were included if these were found, and consistency of results checked for the same study.

Results

We identified 11 population-based studies that had been conducted on hypertension in Ghana between 1973 and 2007. Table 1 shows a summary of the characteristics of the studies and participants as well as methods used for blood pressure measurement. The sample size for individual studies ranged from 287 to 6,900 with a response rate between 53 percent and 97 percent.

A mercury sphygmomanometer was used to assess blood pressure in six studies; an aneuroid sphygmomanometer was used in one study; while electronic monitors were used in four studies. The blood pressure was measured on a single visit in the majority of studies, but blood pressure had been recorded at least twice during the visit in almost all studies and an average value determined. There were four studies involving only rural participants, four studies involving only urban participants and three studies that included both rural and urban or semi-urban participants. The age range of participants varied extensively as shown in Table 1. Table 2 shows the mean blood pressure levels reported from the included studies. The mean SBP ranged between 122.0 and 139.4 mmHg in women and 123.8 mmHg and 132.9 mmHg in men, while mean DBP ranged between 68.8 and 86.4 mmHg in women and 69.2 and 78.4 mmHg in men. In studies with both urban and rural populations, the mean SBP and DBP was higher in the urban than in the rural populations. Table 3 shows the prevalence of hypertension from the individual studies, standardization of hypertension prevalence by age, and the criteria for definition of hypertension. Where available, we reported the levels of detection, treatment and control of hypertension.

Based on the definition of hypertension with a BP >160/95 mmHg, the prevalence of hypertension ranged from 4.5 percent to 16.2 percent whereas using a threshold of BP >140/90 mmHg, the prevalence of hypertension ranged from 19.3 percent to 54.6 percent. For most studies, the prevalence of hypertension was lower in women. The prevalence of hypertension was generally lower in rural compared to urban populations. The prevalence of hypertension reported from Northern Ghana was considerably lower than that reported from other rural populations from more southern parts of Ghana (Kunutsor and Powles, 2009). Hypertension treatment rates ranged from 11.3 percent to 52.5 percent with blood pressure control rates between 1.7 percent and 12.7 percent. The rates of awareness, treatment and control of hypertension were reported to be low in both rural and urban populations. Cappuccio et al (2004) reported the detection, treatment and control rates to be higher in the semiurban compared to rural population. Although higher awareness and treatment rates were reported for older adults, the rates of BP control remained low (Agyemang et al., 2006). There were marked differences in the mean blood pressure values when repeat measurements were taken two weeks after the baseline measurements (Kunutsor and Powles, 2009). The prevalence of hypertension changed from 37.1 percent to 30.3 percent in a study of urban civil servants when repeat measurements taken two weeks after the baseline measurements were considered (Addo et al., 2008).

Temporal trends in mean BP and prevalence of hypertension could not be established conclusively from the available data because of the absence of studies that had conducted serial surveys using the same methodology and population. However, the rural population studied by Addo et al. in 2001 was in the same district previously studied by Pobee in 1973 and showed an increase in the prevalence of hypertension over the period (Addo et al., 2006; Pobee et al., 1977).

The mean BP increased with age in almost all studies where age was reported. The increasing trend in BP with age was less apparent in an earlier study of a rural population (Pobee et al., 1977). Blood pressure was reported to be positively associated with urban dwelling, body mass index, waist circumference, heart rate and a family history of hypertension, parity, and chronic alcohol use (Kunutsor and Powles, 2009; Addo et al., 2006; Amoah, 2003; Agyemang, 2006; Pobee, 1993). A significant and positive relationship was reported between the level of salt intake and both systolic and diastolic blood pressure (Cappuccio et al.,

2006). No significant association was reported between the level of physical activity and hypertension (Addo et al., 2006; Duda et al., 2007).

Examination of the relationship between hypertension and socioeconomic status measured by level of education, income or employment grade was inconclusive. In a study of urban women, there was an inverse relationship between hypertension and education, but there was no demonstrated association with income (Duda et al., 2007). The prevalence of hypertension was, however, higher in civil servants of higher socioeconomic position (Addo et al., 2009).

Table 1.1: Characteristics of studies on hypertension

Author	Year of field work	Study popula-tion	Age range	Sample size	Males/fe-males	Response rate	Preparation	Device	Measures/visits
Pobee [24]	1973	20 rural villages	>=16	1670	809/861	97.5	Seated for 5 to 10 minutes	Mercury sphyg-momanometer	3/1
Pobee [28,50] (1993; 1983)	1975-76	Urban commu-nity	15-64	3745	1635/2100	73	NR	Mercury sphyg-momanometer	NR
Pobee [28,51]	1973	Urban public servants	15-64	6900	5520/1380	91	Seated for 10 minutes	Mercury sphyg-momanometer	2/2
Amoah [26]	1998	Urban and rural communities	25-102 (44.3)	4733	1860/2873	75	Rested for 10 minutes	Mercury sphyg-momanometer	2/1
Addo [25]	2001	4 rural communi-ties	>=18 (42.4)	362	107/255	60-80%	Rested for 10 minutes	Mercury sphyg-momanometer	2/1
Cappuccio [21]	2001-2002	6 semi-urban and 6 rural com-munities	40-75 (54.7)	1013	385/628	53.4	5 minutes rest	Electronic	3/1
Burket [52] (2006)	2002	Rural	>=17 (35.9)	287	NR	NR	NR	Mercury sphyg-momanometer	2/1
Agyemang (2006a,2006b, 2008)	2004	Urban and rural	(35.9)	1431	644/787	82-95	Rested for 5 minutes	Electronic	2/1
Duda [30]	NR	Urban	18-100	1328	NR	NR	NR	Aneuroid sphygmoma-nometer	NR
Addo [23]	2006	Urban civil serv-ants	25-68	1015	615/400	82.7	Ten minutes rest	Electronic	3/2
Kunutsor [20]	2007	Rural	18-65 (37.8)	574	207/367	95.7	NR	Electronic	2/2

NR not reported

Table 1.2: Mean blood pressure levels

Author and year of fieldwork	Study population	Mean SBP (mmHg)			Mean DBP (mmHg)		
		Men	Women	All	Men	Women	All
Pobee , (1973)[24]	Rural	123.8 (19.7)	122.0 (21.0)		69.2 (13.5)	68.8 (12.7)	
Amoah (1998)[26]	Rural and urban	129.0 (22.2)	128.9 (26.7)	128.9 (26.7)	75.1 (13.0)	74.7 (14.1)	74.9 (13.7)
Addo (2001)[25]	Rural	125.4 (20.9)	128.5 (27.6)	127.5 (25.8)	74.5 (14.2)	73.9 (14.4)	74.0 (14.3)
Cappuccio (2001-2002)[21]	Rural and semi-urban	126.3 (24.4)	125.1 (27.0)	125.5 (26.1)	75.8 (13.7)	73.5 (13.5)	74.4 (13.6)
Cappuccio (2001-2002)[21]	Rural			121.5 (25.1)			72.3 (13.2)
Cappuccio (2001-2002)[21]	Semi-urban			129.2 (26.4)			76.2 (13.8)
Agyemang (2004)[22,27]	Rural and urban			130.1 (129.0-131.1)			77.8 (77.1-78.4)
Agyemang (2004)[22,27]	Rural	129.2 (127.1-131.2)	126.3 (124.3-128.3)		75.2 (74.1-76.9)	75.5 (74.3-76.7)	
Agyemang (2004)[22,27]	Urban	132.9 (131.3-134.5)	130.8 (129.1-132.6)		78.4 (77.3-79.5)	80.2 (79.1-81.2)	
Duda[30]	Urban		139.4 (27.5)			86.4 (15.1)	
*Addo, 2006[23]	Urban	131.5 (122.0-144.0)	121.5 (111.3-135.0)	128.5 (117.0-140.5)	80.0 (72.5-89.5)	77.0 (69.0-85.3)	79.0 (71.0-87.5)
Kunutsor, 2007[20]	Rural	124.25 (18.67)	122.07 (22.01)	122.86 (20.88)	69.92 (12.09)	72.11 (12.35)	71.32 (12.29)

*reported median values

Table 1.3: Prevalence of hypertension

Author	Prevalence of hypertension			Detection	Treatment	Control
	All	Men	Women			
Pobee[24]	4.5[a]					
Pobee[28]	13[a]					
Pobee[28,51] (1993, 1971)	7.8[a]	8.9[a]	3.5[a]	24		
Amoah[26]	28.4[b] (16.2)[a]	27.6[b] (14.7)[a]	29.5[b] (17.4)[a]	34	18	4
Cappuccio[21]	28.7	29.9	28.0	22	11.3	2.8
Cappuccio[21]	24.1			16.4	6.9	1.7
Cappuccio[21]	32.9			25.7	14.3	4.4
Addo[25]	25.4 (15.2)[a]			32.3	12.9	2.1
Agyemang[22,27]	29.4			34	28	6.2
Agyemang[22,27]		27.0	27.0	26.6 (34.8)[d]	23.4 (29.3)[d]	4.7 (7.6)[d]
Agyemang[22,27]		33.4	28.9	27.2 (44.2)[d]	22.8 (34.9)[d]	5.1 (7.0)[d]
Duda[30]			54.6		52.5	4.4
Addo[23]	37.1 (30.3)[c] (27.4)[b]	31.7[c]	28.0[c]	54.1	31.3	12.7
Burket[52]	32.8	39.4	30.7			
Kunutsor	19.3					

Study population: Pobee[24] Rural; Pobee[28] Urban community; Pobee[28,51] Urban public servants; Amoah[26] Rural and urban; Cappuccio[21] Rural and semi-urban; Cappuccio[21] Rural; Cappuccio[21] Semi-urban; Addo[25] Rural; Agyemang[22,27] Rural and urban; Agyemang[22,27] Rural; Agyemang[22,27] Urban.

a hypertension defined by WHO criteria (160/95)

b prevalence age-standardised to new world standard population

c prevalence defined by readings from two visits two weeks apart

d values in brackets are the rates for women

Discussion

This review of population-based studies conducted on hypertension in Ghana identified a number of studies conducted since 1973 involving rural as well as urban adults. There were variations in the criteria used in selecting participants and methods applied in blood pressure measurements in the studies. The age structure of the different populations also varied extensively and very few studies provided age-standardised data, thus limiting the ability to directly compare the results between studies. Almost all studies had based the classification of hypertension on blood pressure readings taken at a single visit with the possibility of overestimating the prevalence of hypertension and there was very little information on temporal trends in the prevalence of hypertension. Despite these limitations, there was clear evidence of differences in prevalence, with urban areas consistently having a higher prevalence of hypertension. The prevalence of hypertension among urban populations in Ghana was comparable to that reported from Europe and North America (Kearney et al, 2004; Wolf-Maier et al., 2003).

In the recent rural studies the prevalence of hypertension was lowest in a study from a rural area in northern Ghana which is more economically disadvantaged than the other rural areas studied. The prevalence of hypertension increased with age in almost all studies, contrary to earlier reports from some rural African studies where little or no rise in blood pressure with age had been observed among nomads, rural agricultural males and indigenous people (Poulter et al., 1984; Shaper et al., 1969; Sever et al,. 1980). Hypertension was positively associated with body mass index, waist circumference, pulse rate, excessive alcohol consumption, salt intake and a positive family history of hypertension.

Most of the studies did not report the association between hypertension and physical activity, and the relationship with socioeconomic status was inconclusive. The rates of detection, treatment and control were low in all studies that had reported these and were reported to be even lower in rural areas than urban areas.

The findings of this review have important public health implications. First, an increased burden of hypertension should be expected in Ghana in the absence of effective hypertension prevention programmes. This is especially true given the rapid rate of urbanisation, and increased life expectancy with increased access to health care. Secondly, complications such as strokes, heart failure and renal failure are undoubtedly going to become more apparent if the current low levels of detection, treatment and control of hypertension persist, and this would certainly place a further weight on the already overburdened health infrastructure. Prevention and control of hypertension in Ghana is thus imperative.

Primary prevention of hypertension provides a good opportunity to interrupt and prevent the continuing costly management of hypertension and its complications (National High Blood Pressure Education Program, 1993). This can be accomplished by the complementary application of strategies targeting the general population with the objective of achieving a downward shift in the distribution of blood pressure, as well as targeting individuals and groups at higher risk of developing hypertension (National High Blood Pressure Education Program, 1993; Rose, 1985; Whelton et al., 2002). It has been suggested that prevention strategies applied early in life, provide the greatest long-term potential for avoiding the precursors that lead to hypertension and for reducing the overall burden of blood pressure-related complications in the community (Whelton et al., 2002). Engaging in regular aerobic physical activity, maintaining a normal body mass index, reduction of dietary salt intake to no more than 100mmol/day, moderation in alcohol intake, maintaining adequate intake of dietary potassium, and consumption of a diet rich in fruits and vegetables and in low-fat dairy products, but with a reduced content of saturated and total fat have been shown to be beneficial in the prevention of hypertension (Whelton et al., 2002; Appel et al., 1997; Sacks et al., 2001).

A community programme in the Ashanti Region to establish the feasibility of salt reduction as a way of reducing blood pressure showed that a reduction in average salt intake led to a small but important reduction in blood pressure (Cappucio et al., 2006). It is important for lifestyle and dietary habits that promote the primary prevention of hypertension and cardiovascular disease to be encouraged among the entire Ghanaian population, including the youth and children. The maintenance of ideal body weight through reduced fat and total calorie intake, an increase in physical activity as well as a reduction in dietary sodium intake should be emphasised. Information on hypertension should be disseminated through the appropriate media. These could be achieved through mass media campaigns, engagement of the lay public and non-governmental organisations in dissemination of information on hypertension and production of simple and easy to read booklets on hypertension. The information should address what hypertension is, how it is diagnosed and managed, and the potential complications that could occur when left uncontrolled. In educating people, is important to emphasise the usual absence of symptoms, need for long term therapy and monitoring, and the importance of lifestyle and diet in the primary prevention of hypertension. School and work-based health education programmes could be beneficial. The population strategy should be complemented with targeting of preventive efforts at those considered to be at high risk of developing hypertension.

In this effort it is important to include early detection through screening programs as well as appropriate treatment and control of hypertension when detected. Limited resources, poor delivery of care at community health centres, unreliable drug supply and unreliable equipment to measure blood pressure in some health facilities, unavailability of basic investigations, lack of assessment of target organ damage, risk stratification and global cardiovascular risk reduction are reported to be major obstacles to providing better detection and treatment of hypertension in sub-Saharan Africa (Thorogood et al., 2007; Seedat and Rosenthal, 2006; Rayner et al., 2007). These hurdles could possibly be surmounted in Ghana if the government has hypertension prevention high on the agenda and allocates adequate resources to achieving this. It is necessary to develop guidelines for hypertension management in Ghana, targeted at all health professionals in both public and private sectors. These guidelines should reflect realistic objectives that can be applied widely in the Ghanaian context. Despite very effective anti-hypertensive therapies and data from clinical trials demonstrating that lowering blood pressure reduces cardiovascular and renal complications, a significant proportion of people with known hypertension from both developed and developing countries have blood pressure exceeding recommended levels (Chobanian, 2001). There could be various possible explanations for the low treatment and poor control of hypertension in SSA. These include scarce resources, lack of patient education, and poor organization of the healthcare systems. Unaffordable drug prices have been reported to be the major cause of non-compliance with hypertension medication in Ghana (Ohene Buabeng et al., 2004). It is reported however, that even in healthcare systems with generous resources, control of blood pressure is often unsatisfactory (Okano et al., 1997).

This suggests that although hypertension control is probably dependent on the availability and affordability of medication, there are other factors that play a role and these need to be investigated and appropriate measures taken to address them. Although rural Ghanaians rarely buy ready-made and processed foods, urban populations continue to face a rapid influx of restaurants and fast-food joints, most of which serve foods heavily laden with salt and fat. Processed canned foods with high salt content are also more readily available and increasingly becoming more affordable. It is important for the health sector to liaise with the food sector to address the issue of hidden salts and fats in processed foods and determine how these could be effectively regulated.

It may require voluntary agreements with the food industry or policies from central government mandating reductions in salt and fat in these foods. Recommendations by health professionals to modify diets or to increase physical activity will be hampered by lack of healthier and affordable food choices, and by lack of safe, attractive places to be physically active (Pearson et al., 2003). Environmental and legislative interventions that facilitate widespread adoption of healthy lifestyles, and the development of policies to strengthen primary healthcare systems will be crucial for the prevention and control of high blood pressure and stroke (Mensah, 2008).

Conclusions

The limited number of population-based studies with age-standardised data that allow direct comparison between studies, the heterogeneity of the methods and the absence of data on temporal trends underscore the importance of obtaining more data using rigorous methods to inform policy and practice on hypertension and cardiovascular disease in Ghana. The relatively limited evidence available suggests an increasing prevalence of hypertension in both urban and rural populations but more so in urban groups associated with increasing body mass index, salt intake and other risk factors as well as poor detection, treatment and control rates. These findings certainly raise important concerns. Cardiovascular disease and its major risk factors such as hypertension undoubtedly compete with other conditions such as malaria, HIV/AIDS, maternal and infant mortality for the limited resources. However, uncontrolled hypertension potentially increases the risk of developing complications of hypertension with grave consequences on the individual, family and the entire society. Ignoring the need to institute effective prevention strategies now will certainly result in a greater burden with increased challenges in the near future.

References

Addo, J., Amoah, A.G, Koram, K.A. (2006). The changing patterns of hypertension in Ghana: a study of four rural communities in the Ga District. *Ethnicity and Disease*, 16:894-899.

Addo, J., Smeeth, L., Leon, D.A. (2007). Hypertension in sub-saharan Africa: a systematic review. *Hypertension.* 50:1012-1018.

Addo, J., Smeeth, L, Leon, D.A. (2008). Prevalence, detection, management, and control of hypertension in Ghanaian civil servants. *Ethnicity and Disease.*18:505-511.

Addo, .J, Smeeth, L., Leon, D.A. (2009). Socioeconomic position and hypertension: a study of urban civil servants in Ghana. *J Epidemiol Community Health.*

Agyemang, C. (2006). Rural and urban differences in blood pressure and hypertension in Ghana, West Africa. *Public Health.* 120:525-533.

Agyemang, C., Bruijnzeels, M.A., Owusu-Dabo, E. (2006). Factors associated with hypertension awareness, treatment, and control in Ghana, West Africa. *J Hum Hypertens.* 20:67-71.

Agyemang, C. and Owusu-Dabo, E. 92008). Prehypertension in the Ashanti region of Ghana, West Africa: an opportunity for early prevention of clinical hypertension. *Public Health.* 122:19-24.

Amoah, A.G. (2003). Hypertension in Ghana: a cross-sectional community prevalence study in greater Accra. *Ethn Dis.* 13:310-315.

Appel, L.J., Moore, T.J., Obarzanek, E., Vollmer, W.M., Svetkey, L.P., Sacks, F.M. et al. (1997). A clinical trial of the effects of dietary patterns on blood pressure. DASH Collaborative Research Group. *N Engl J Med.* 336:1117-1124.

Beaglehole R. (2001). Global cardiovascular disease prevention: time to get serious. *Lancet.* 358:661-663.

Bonita, R. W.R. and Douglas, K. (2001). The WHO STEP wise approach to NCD risk factor surveillance. In: McQueen and Puska P(eds). *Global Behavioural Risk Factor Surveillance.* Cordrecht :Kluwer.

Brown, M.J. (2006). Hypertension and ethnic group. *British Medical Journal,* 332:833-836.

Burket, B.A. (2006). Blood pressure survey in two communities in the Volta region, Ghana, West Africa. *Ethn Dis.* 16:292-294.

Cappuccio, F.P., Micah, F.B., Emmett, L., Kerry, S.M., Antwi, S., Martin-Peprah, R. et al.9 2004). Prevalence, detection, management, and control of hypertension in Ashanti, West Africa. *Hypertension.* 43:1017-1022.

Cappuccio, F.P., Kerry, S.M., Micah, F.B., Plange-Rhule, J., and Eastwood, J.B. (2006). A community programme to reduce salt intake and blood pressure in Ghana [ISRCTN88789643]. *BMC Public Health.* 6:13.

Chobanian, A.V. Control of hypertension--an important national priority. (2001). *N Engl J Med*. 345:534-535.

Chobanian, A.V., Bakris, G.L., Black, H.R., Cushman, W.C., Green, L.A., Izzo, J.L, Jr. et al. (2003). The Seventh Report of the Joint National Committee on Prevention, Detection, Evaluation, and Treatment of High Blood Pressure: the JNC 7 report. *Jama*. 289:2560-2572.

Duda, R.B., Kim, M.P., Darko, R., Adanu, R.M., Seffah, J., Anarf,i J.K. et al. (2007). Results of the Women's Health Study of Accra: assessment of blood pressure in urban women. *Int J Cardiol*. 117:115-122.

Ezzati, M. V.H.S., Lawes, C.M., Leach, R., James,P.T., Lopez, A.D., Rodgers, A. and Murray, C.J. (2005). Rethinking the "Diseases of Affluence" Paradigm: Global Patterns of Nutritional Risks in Relation to Economic Development. *PLoS Med*. 2(5):e133.

Kearney, P.M., Whelton, M., Reynolds, K., Whelton, P.K. and He, J.92004). Worldwide prevalence of hypertension: a systematic review. *J Hypertens*. 22:11-19.

Kearney ,P.M, Whelton, M., Reynolds, K., Muntner, P., Whelton, P.K. and He J. (2005). Global burden of hypertension: analysis of worldwide data. *Lancet*. 365:217-223.

Khor, G.L. (2001). Cardiovascular epidemiology in the Asia-Pacific region. *Asia Pac J Clin Nutr*. 10:76-80.

Kunutsor, S., and Powles, J. (2009). Descriptive epidemiology of blood pressure in a rural adult population in Northern Ghana. *Rural Remote Health*. 9:1095.

Mathers, C.D. and Loncar, D. (2006). Projections of global mortality and burden of disease from 2002 to 2030. *PLoS Med*. 3:e442.

Mendis, S., Yach, D., Bengoa, R., Narvaez, D., Zhang, X. (2003). Research gap in cardiovascular disease in developing countries. *Lancet*. 361:2246-2247.

Mensah, G.A. (2008). Epidemiology of stroke and high blood pressure in Africa. *Heart*. 94:697-705.

Ministry of Health(MOH) (2005). The Ghana Health Sector 2006 Programme of Work. Accra: MOH.

National High Blood Pressure Education Program Working Group.(1993). report on primary prevention of hypertension. *Arch Intern Med*. 153:186-208.

Ohene Buabeng, K., Matowe, L. and Plange-Rhule, J. (2004). Unaffordable drug prices: the major cause of non-compliance with hypertension medication in Ghana. *J Pharm Pharm Sci*. 7:350-352.

Okano, G.J., Rascati, K.L., Wilson, J.P., Remund, D.D., Grabenstein, J.D., and Brixner D.I.(1997). Patterns of antihypertensive use among patients in the US Department of Defense database initially prescribed an angiotensin-converting enzyme inhibitor or calcium channel blocker. *Clin Ther*. 19:1433-1445; discussion 1424-1435.

Pearson, T.A., Bazzarre , T.L., Daniels, S.R., Fair, J.M., Fortmann, S.P., Franklin, B.A. et al. (2003). American Heart Association guide for improving cardiovascular health at the community level: a statement for public health practitioners, healthcare providers, and health policy makers from the American Heart Association Expert Panel on Population and Prevention Science. *Circulation*. 107:645-651.

Pobee, J.O.M. (1983). Epidemiological report from West Africa. In Gross F, Strasser T, eds. Mild Hypertension: Recent Advances. New York, Raven Press. 33-53.

Pobee, J.O. (1993). Community-based high blood pressure programs in sub-Saharan Africa. *Ethn Dis*. 3 Suppl:S38-45.

Pobee J.O., Larbi, E.B., Belcher, D.W., Wurapa, F.K., Dodu, S.R. (1977). Blood pressure distribution in a rural Ghanaian population. *Trans R Soc Trop Med Hyg*. 71:66-72.

Pobee, J.O., Larbi, E.B., Dodu, S.R., Pisa, Z., and Strasser T. (1979). Is systemic hypertension a problem in Ghana? *Trop Doct*. 9:89-92.

Poulter, N., Khaw, K.T., Hopwood, B.E., Mugambi, M., Pear,t W.S., Rose, G. et al. (1984a). Blood pressure and associated factors in a rural Kenyan community. *Hypertension*. 6:810-813.

Poulter, N., Khaw, K.T., Hopwood, B.E., Mugambi, M., Peart, W.S., Rose, G. et al. (1984b). Blood pressure and its correlates in an African tribe in urban and rural environments. *J Epidemiol Community Health*. 38:181-185.

Rayner, B., Blockman, M., Baines, D., Trinder, Y. (2007). A survey of hypertensive practices at two community health centres in Cape Town. *S Afr Med J*. 97:280-284.

Rodgers, A., Ezzati, M., Vander Hoorn, S., Lopez, A.D., Lin, R.B,. Murray. C.J. (2004). Distribution of major health risks: findings from the Global Burden of Disease study. *PLoS Med*. 1:e27.

Rose, G. (1985). Sick individuals and sick populations. *Int J Epidemiol*. 14:32-38.

Sacks, F.M., Svetkey, L.P., Vollmer, W.M., Appel, L.J., Bray, G.A., Harsha, D. et al. (2001). Effects on blood pressure of reduced dietary sodium and the Dietary Approaches to Stop Hypertension (DASH) diet. DASH-Sodium Collaborative Research Group. *N Engl J Med*. 344:3-10.

Seedat, Y.K., Rosenthal, T. (2006). Meeting the challenges of hypertension in sub-Saharan Africa. *Cardiovasc J S Afr*. 17:47-48.

Sever, P.S., Gordon, D., Peart, W.S., Beighton, P. (1980). Blood-pressure and its correlates in urban and tribal Africa. *Lancet*. 2:60-64.

Shaper, A.G., Wright, D.H., Kyobe, J. (1969). Blood pressure and body build in three nomadic tribes of northern Kenya. *East Afr Med J*. 46:273-281.

Singh, R.B., Suh, I.L., Singh, V.P., Chaithiraphan, S., Laothavorn, P., Sy, R.G. et al. (2000). Hypertension and stroke in Asia: prevalence, control and strategies in developing countries for prevention. *J Hum Hypertens.* 14:749-763.

Thorogood, M., Connor, M.D., Hundt, G.L. and Tollman, S.M. (2007). Understanding and managing hypertension in an African sub-district: a multidisciplinary approach. *Scand J Public Health Suppl.* 69:52-59.

Unwin ,N., Setel, P., Rashid, S., Mugusi, F., Mbanya, J.C., Kitange. H. et al. (2001) Noncommunicable diseases in sub-Saharan Africa: where do they feature in the health research agenda? *Bull World Health Organ.* 79:947-953.

Vorster, H.H. (2002). The emergence of cardiovascular disease during urbanisation of Africans. *Public Health Nutr.* 5:239-243.

Whelton, P.K., He, J., Appel, L.J., Cutler, J.A., Havas, S., Kotchen, T.A. et al. (2002). Primary prevention of hypertension: clinical and public health advisory from The National High Blood Pressure Education Program. *Jama.* 288:1882-1888.

Wiredu, E.K.and Nyame P.K. (2001). Stroke-related mortality at Korle Bu Teaching Hospital, Accra,Ghana. *East Afr Med J.* 78:180-184.

Wolf-Maier, K., Cooper, R.S., Banegas, J.R., Giampaoli, S., Hense, H.W., Joffres M, et al. (2003). Hypertension prevalence and blood pressure levels in 6 European countries, Canada, and the United States. *Jama.* 289:2363-2369.

Yach, D., Leeder, S.R., Bell, J.and Kistnasamy, B. (2005). Global chronic diseases. *Science.* 307:317.

Yusuf ,S., Reddy, S., Ounpuu, S., Anand, S. (2001). Global burden of cardiovascular diseases: part I: general considerations, the epidemiologic transition, risk factors, and impact of urbanization. *Circulation.* 104:2746-2753.

Chapter 2

Stroke in Ghana: a systematic literature review

Olutobi Sanuade and Charles Agyemang

Introduction

Stroke is the second leading cause of disability worldwide, following dementia (WHO, 2012). The World Health Organization (WHO) estimates that globally, 15 million people suffer from stroke every year. Out of this number, about 6 million people die and another five million people are left permanently disabled. In sub-Saharan Africa (SSA), cardiovascular disease is projected to eclipse infectious diseases as the leading cause of mortality, morbidity and premature loss of healthy life expectancy, and many of these losses will come from stroke (Kengne and Anderson 2006). Stroke is associated with the greatest likelihood of reported severe disability in the population (Adamson, Beswick and Ebrahim 2004). More importantly, stroke is associated with more individual domains of disability (cognitive, behavioural, physical) compared with other conditions and might be considered as the most common cause of complex disability (Adamson, Beswick and Ebrahim, 2004). Compared with other diseases, stroke is a major health problem that can cause multiple or concurrent disabilities in an individual. The disabilities associated with stroke can influence all dimensions of life, including the simplest self-care tasks (Bury, 1982; Adamson, Beswick and Ebrahim, 2004).

In Ghana, stroke morbidity is projected to go up as a result of urbanization, poor socio-economic status and the change in the demographic structure of the population. The country is becoming more urbanized, the lifestyles are also changing, thereby providing the conditions for more stroke morbidity. Of Ghana's total population, 50.9 percent were living in urban areas in 2010 -- Ghana Statistical Service, (2012). 2010 Population and Housing Census -- Summary Report of Final Results. Accra: GSS. p. 3.) Although stroke can occur at any age, it is a condition that primarily affects elderly persons. Hence, the number of stroke survivors may continue to increase as the number of elderly persons increases. It is projected that the number of people who will be aged 60 years and above in Ghana, which is 4 percent as at 2012, will more than double by 2025 (Population and Reference Bureau, 2012). This projected demographic shift may seriously increase stroke-induced disability in the country, with serious implications on the quality of life of stroke survivors.

The stroke burden has been increasing in Ghana (Gould et al. 1995; de-Graft Aikins, 2007). With the emerging elderly population in Ghana, the incidence of stroke in the country may continue to grow at an alarming rate if serious measures are not put in place to curtail this (Darkwa, 1999). Despite this projection, there is dearth of literature on the epidemiology of stroke in Ghana. This study intends to undertake a summary of the current knowledge on the stroke burden in Ghana, identify gaps in the literature and provide indications for future research in the country.

Methods

A search of MEDLINE and Google Scholar from 1 January 1900 to 31 May 2013 was conducted on stroke in Ghana. Using the MeSH term "stroke in Ghana" provided 36 studies, however, eight entries were relevant to stroke. The same search term was entered in Google Scholar and three additional entries were retrieved, thus providing a total of 11 articles published on stoke in Ghana from the beginning of the 20th century until 31st May 2013. Studies were included if they focused on stroke in Ghana and were published within the stipulated period. However, studies which were published on stroke in other countries or sub-Saharan Africa were not included in this study. The retrieved data were analysed by dividing them into different sections in order to provide clear information on the stroke burden in Ghana.

Description of the studies

Many of the studies on stroke in Ghana were carried out in the hospital environment and most of them were done at Korle-Bu Teaching Hospital (Table 1). In terms of design, a larger proportion of these studies were retrospective in nature. The sample sizes on stroke burden ranges from 19 to 9,760 participants. The study with the largest sample size examined stroke mortality for a five-year period. Most of the studies focused on stroke mortality and stroke rehabilitation.

Stroke mortality and morbidity in Ghana

Since the first case of stroke was recorded at the Korle-Bu Teaching Hospital (KBTH) in the early 1920s, there has been an increase in stroke mortality and morbidity in Ghana (Agyei-Mensah and de-Graft Aikins, 2010). In the first study on mortality from cardiovascular disease in the then Gold Coast, from 1921 to 1953, 73 deaths out of 3,645 autopsies (2 percent) were due to stroke (Edington,1954). More recent data suggest that stroke has become a major cause of morbidity and mortality (Nyame et al. 1994). Between 1972 and 1981, the overall incidence of stroke as a cause of death at KBTH was 11 percent (Anim, 1984). The same proportion of stroke death was also recorded between 1994 and 1998 at KBTH (Wiredu and Nyame, 2001). Also, a recent study of stroke morbidity at Komfo Anokye Teaching Hospital (KATH) from January 2006 to December 2007 shows that stroke constitutes 13.2 percent of all medical adult deaths (Agyemang et al. 2012). In terms of stroke severity, a larger proportion of stroke survivors in Ghana experience mild and moderate stroke. In a prospective study of 160 stroke survivors at KBTH, 48.7 percent had mild stroke, 33.8 percent had moderate stroke and 17.5 percent had severe stroke (Akpalu & Nyame, 2009). The onset of stroke in Ghana is shown to occur early in the morning. For instance, the peak onsets is between 0600 h and 1000 h and there is no significant difference in time of onset between men and women or hypertensive and non-hypertensive stroke patients (Roberts, Opare-Sem and Acheampong, 1994).

Risk factors of stroke

The main risk factors of stroke reported in other countries were also reported in Ghana. Hypertension, diabetes, and obesity constitute important associated factors of stroke in Ghana (Agyei-Mensah and de-Graft Aikins, 2010; Wiredu and Nyame, 2001; Agyemang et al., 2012). Another risk factor of stroke which is not commonly known is plasma level of homocysteine. A study has shown that there is a significant relationship between a high level of homocysteine and stroke (Akpalu and Nyame, 2009).

Table 2.1: **Key Published literature on stroke in Ghana**

Location	First Author	Year pub-lished	Setting	Design	Sample size	Male: female	Age (years)	Key findings
KBTH	Edington GM [11]	1954	Hospital	Retrospective	3645	-	-	Stroke accounted for 2 percent of all deaths at KBTH from 1921 to 1953.
KBTH	Roberts MA [17]	1994	-	Prospective	68	-	-	The peak onsets of stroke in Ghana is between 0600 h and 1000 h and time of onsets does not differ for men and women.
KBTH	Nyame PK [12]	1998	Hospital	Retrospective	1003	-	-	907 of those clinically diagnosed as stroke were proven to have suffered stroke using CT scan. No diagnosis was made in 56 of the patients.
KBTH	Wiredu EK [14]	2001	Hospital (urban) subtypes of stroke	Cross-sectional	9760	1.2:1	50-59 for HS, 60-69 for CI	Stroke accounted for 11 percent of autopsies carried out at KBTH from 1994 to 1998.
Accra	Obajimi MO [19]	2002	Hospital (urban) subtypes of stroke	Retrospective	1172	-	55.7	CT patterns of intracranial infarcts in Ghanaians show that the infarcts' diagnosis appearance was a wedge shaped hypodensity within the brain parenchyma and which is often found in parietal lobe.
KBTH and 37 Military Hospital	Hamzat TK [23]	2008	Hospital	Ex post facto	50	-	-	The prescription of cane can help in restoration of balance functions and social participation of stroke survivors.
KBTH	Akpalu AK [16]	2009	Hospital	Prospective	160	1.4:1	57.3	A significant relationship exists between a high level of homocysteine and stroke. The mean homocysteine level in stroke cases was higher than the one measured in controls.

Location	First Author	Year published	Setting	Design	Sample size	Male: female	Age (years)	Key findings
KBTH	Bello AI [20]	2009	Hospital	Experimental	19	-	-	Electromyographic-triggered neuromuscular electrical muscle stimulation can help in better functional and hand recovery of stroke survivors during recovery stage.
KATH	Agyemang C [15]	2012	Hospital	Retrospective	1050	1:0.96	63.7	Stroke accounted for 13.2% of all medical adult deaths at KATH from 2006 to 2007 and the stroke case fatality rate within this period was 43.2% at 28 days.
KBTH	Bello AI [21]	2012	Hospital	Cross-sectional	80	-	56.7	Joint range of motion, level of spasticity and disability were the main determinants of static balance among stroke survivors.
Accra, Kumasi and Eastern Region	Amosun SL [22]	2013	Hospital	Descriptive Mixed-method interview)	200	-	53.7	The perception of stroke survivors in terms of their ability to take up and participate in daily activities can facilitate stroke recovery process. However, stigmatization can slow than this process.

HS= Haemorrhagic stroke, CI=Cerebral infarction, IS= Ischemic stroke KBTH= Korle-Bu Teaching Hospital KATH= Komfo Anokye Teaching Hospital
CT= Computerised tomography

Sex Differences

In general, the studies show that a higher proportion of stroke survivors are males (Wiredu & Nyame 2001; Akpalu & Nyame 2009). Also, in terms of mortality, stroke deaths is higher among males than among females in all age group up to 60-69 years. However, at older ages, mortality is higher among females (Wiredu & Nyame 2001). In Accra, females have higher relative risk of stroke deaths than males although males are more likely to die from haemorrhagic stroke than females (Wiredu & Nyame 2001). On the other hand, in Kumasi, at KATH, the relative risk of death from stroke was lower for females than males (Agyemang et al. 2012). Another study shows that female admissions and deaths (8.6 percent and 24.6 percent respectively) in Ghana far outnumbered male admissions and deaths (1.8 percent and 20 percent respectively) (Agyei-Mensah & de-Graft Aikins 2010).

Types of stroke

Generally, more than half of stroke in Ghana are haemorrhagic. Several studies on the pattern of stroke in Accra have shown that 60% to 90% of strokes are haemorrhagic (Binder 1961; Nyame et al. 1994; Wiredu & Nyame 2001). Another study shows that about 52.9% of stroke are haemorrhagic (Obajimi et al. 2002). However, in 2009, more than 60% of the stroke identified at KBTH were cerebral infarction (Akpalu & Nyame 2009). In general, many of the studies show that haemorrhagic stroke is more common than cerebral infarction in Ghana.

Age

Age is seen as one of the risk factors of stroke. The age of stroke onset vary from one country to another and can also vary within a country. Generally, the mean age of stroke onset in Accra is lower than that of Kumasi. The mean age of stroke onset in Ghana vary from 56.7 years in Accra to 63.7 years in Kumasi (Akpalu & Nyame 2009; Obajimi et al. 2002). Also, the peak age of haemorrhagic stroke in Accra is 50-59 years and 60-69 years for cerebral infarction (Wiredu & Nyame 2001). In essence, the age at death for haemorrhaguc stroke is lower than that of cerebral infarction.

Stroke Admissions

Stroke is rising fast as an increasing proportion of medical admissions in Ghana. Between 1960 and 1968, stroke accounted for 8 percent of medical admissions and 10.4 percent by 1972 (Agyei-Mensah and de-Graft Aikins, 2010). In terms of stroke admission, many of the stroke survivors are admitted within 48 hours of stroke onsets. For instance, about 56.3 percent of stroke survivors at KBTH were admitted within the first 24 hours and 18.8 percent within 48 hours (Akpalu and Nyame, 2009).

Case fatality rate

In Accra, about 69 percent of stroke deaths in 2001 occurred in less than 24 hours after the onset of the disease (Wiredu and Nyame 2001). In Kumasi, the case fatality rate of stroke was 5.7 percent at 24 hours, 32.7 percent at 7 days and 43.2 percent at 28 days (Agyemang et al. 2012). While most of the stroke deaths occurred within 24 hours in Accra, majority of deaths occurred in Kumasi occurred within the first seven days of admissions (Wiredu and Nyame, 2001; Agyemang et al. 2012).

Stroke rehabilitation

Many studies have been done on stroke rehabilitation in Ghana. Studies have shown that electromyographic-triggered neuromuscular electrical muscle stimulation of stroke survivors, perceived ability participation in daily activities, and social acceptance can facilitate rehabilitation of stroke survivors in Ghana. For instance, electromyographic-triggered neuromuscular electrical muscle stimulation, low disability and spasticity can help in functional and hand recovery of stroke survivors (Bello, Rockson and Olaogun, 2009; Bello, Oduro and Adjei, 2012). Further, stroke survivors' perception in their ability to take up and participate in daily activities can help in their recovery process (Amosun, Nyante and Wiredu, 2013). On the other hand, stigmatization can slow down the recovery process. Two types of stigma have been identified in this regard: the felt stigma and the enacted stigma (Amosun, Nyante and Wiredu, 2013). While enacted stigma manifests as discrimination against the stigmatized person which is imposed by others, felt stigma is the fear of enacted stigma experienced by stigmatized person. It has been shown that felt stigma reduces stroke survivor participation in normal life experiences (Amosun, Nyante and Wiredu, 2013). Further, prescription of canes for stroke survivors can be useful in the stroke rehabilitation process most especially if the focus of rehabilitation is to restore balance functions and social participation of stroke survivors (Hamzat and Kobiri, 2008).

Discussion

Generally, stroke constitutes more than one-tenth of all causes of deaths in Ghana. The data also suggest increasing stroke incidence in the country. This is contrary to what happens in high-income countries where the incidence of stroke is decreasing (WHO, 2012). The findings show that many of the stroke survivors in Ghana experience mild and moderate stroke. The implication of this is that since many of the hospitals in Ghana only admit people with severe stroke due to insufficient bed and experts, those with mild and moderate stroke may have to be cared for at home and this may make rehabilitation very challenging.

The main risk factor of stroke in Ghana is hypertension and it is projected to increase in Ghana due to urbanization. However, few facilities are available for the detection and management of hypertension in the country (Plange-Rhule et al., 1999; Agyemang et al., 2012). Specifically, the high incidence of haemorrhagic stroke among the young adult in Ghana may be due to the increase in high blood pressure among these group (Anim and Kofi, 1989). It is therefore important to pay particular attention to reducing high blood pressure in Ghana in order to reduce stroke burden (Agyemang et al., 2012). Since hyperhomocysteine is also modifiable risk factor, reducing this can also reduce the burden of stroke in Ghana.

There have been different conclusions on the impact of sex on stroke. While some studies show that females have a higher risk of stroke deaths, other studies reveal the contrary. Since it is difficult to calculate the rate of stroke incidence by sex, due to the absence of population at risk, it may be difficult to reach a conclusion in terms of the impact of sex on the stroke burden in Ghana. There is a need for population-based studies in Ghana in order to determine which sex is more at risk.

In terms of admissions, those who are usually admitted in Ghana hospitals are those who experience severe stroke cases because of lack of beds and experts (Hamzat and Kobiri, 2008). Since studies have shown that many of the stroke survivors are admitted within 48 hours of stroke onset. This means that late presentation to hospital may not be an explanation for high case fatality rate of stroke in Ghana. One plausible explanation for the high case fatality rate in the country may be the inadequate health care system which is crippled by inadequate human and financial resources (de-Graft Aikins, 2007).

Since felt stigma among stroke survivors has been identified as hindrance to participation in normal life, there is need for the physiotherapists and providers of traditional rehabilitation to address this felt stigma in order to enhance stroke rehabilitation in Ghana. Despite the stroke prognosis, only the most severely affected stroke patients are admitted in Ghana due to lack of beds and scarcity of experts (Moris, 2011). As a result, there is a three-year collaboration of health professionals from Wessex, UK and Accra, Ghana in order to improvestroke care through better day-to-day management and multidisciplinary work in order to improve stroke care in changing day-to-day management and improve multidisciplinary work. (Moris, 2011). The UK group had made three visits to Ghana. The major achievement is that the Ghanaian team now meets every week and indictes the acute stroke checklist which is being piloted. This indicates the potential for stroke care improvement and management in Ghana. Hence, the collaboration of health professionals from UK and Accra needs to be taken seriously to improve stroke care in its many dimensions, from acute positioning to neurorehabilitation, and from managing patient expectations of recovery to delivering palliative care.

Generally, many of the studies on stroke in Ghana were done in Accra and Kumasi, which are the two most developed cities in the country. There is a need for population-based data that will capture all the regions in Ghana in order to determine the regional pattern of the disease for appropriate policies to be put in place. Also, there is a need for studies on how stroke patients are cared for at home after discharge from hospital and the impact this has on their families.

Limitations

The majority of the publications were hospital-based studies done at Korle-Bu Teaching Hospital (KBTH), Accra, and Komfo Anokye Teaching Hospital (KATH), Kumasi. There is lack of data on stroke in other regions in Ghana. No community-based study has been done on stroke and the few studies done are indicative of paucity of data on stroke in the country. Since most of the publications are hospital-based studies, it is difficult to generalize the findings to the whole country.

Conclusions

This review discusses the burden of stroke in Ghana. Even though the stroke burden is projected to increase due to urbanization and an increase in ageing population, there is a dearth of literature on stroke in Ghana. Currently, there is no community-based study on stroke burden in Ghana. In order to understand the stroke burden, there is an urgent need for population-based data which would help to trigger effective primary, secondary and tertiary prevention strategies.

References

Adamson, J, Beswick, A & Ebrahim, S. (2004). 'Is stroke the most common cause of disability?', Journal of Stroke and Cerebrovascular Diseases, vol.13, no.4, pp.171-177.

Agyei-Mensah, S & de-Graft Aikins, A (2010). 'Epidemiological Transition and the double burden of disease in Accra, Ghana', Journal of Urban Health: Bulletin of the New York Academy of medicine, vol.87, no.5, pp.879-897.

Agyemang, C, Attah-Adejepong, G, Owusu-Dabo, E, de-Graft Aikins,A, Addo, J, Edusei A.K, Nkum, BC, and Ogedegbe, O (2012). 'Stroke in Ashanti Region of Ghana', *Ghana medical Journal*, vol.45, no.2, pp.12-17.

Akpalu, A.K, and Nyame P.K. (2009). 'Plasma homocysteine as a risk factor for strokes in Ghanaian Adults', *Ghana Medical Journal*, vol.43, no.4, pp.157-163.

Amosun, S.L., Nyante, G.G., and Wiredu, E.K. (2013). 'Perceived and experienced restrictions in participation and autonomy among adult survivors of stroke in Ghana', *Afr Health Sci.*, vol.13, no.1, pp.24–31.

Anim, J.T. (1984). 'Mortality from stroke and other complications of hypertension in Accra', *West African Journal of Medical*, Vol.3, No.2, pp. 85-90.

Anim, J.I. and Kofi, A.D. (1989). 'Hypertension, cerebral vascular changes and stroke in Ghana: a cerebral atherosclerosis and stroke', *East Afr Med J*, vol.66, no.7, pp.468-75.

Bello, A.I., Rockson, B.E. and Olaogun M.O. (2009). 'The effects of electromyographic-triggered neuromuscular electrical muscle stimulation on the functional hand recovery among stroke survivors', Afr J Med Med Sci, vol.38, no.2, pp.185-191.

Bello, A.I., Oduro, R. and Adjei, D.N. (2012). 'Influence of clinical and demographic factors on static balance among stroke survivors', Afr J Med Med Sci, vol.414, pp.393-398.

Binder, E. (1961). 'Cardiovascular disease in Accra (Ghana) as suggested by analysis of post-mortem records', W. Afr. Med. J, vol.10, pp.158-170.

Bury, M. (1982). 'Chronic illness as biographical disruption', Sociology of Health and Illness, vol.4, no.2, pp.167-182.

Darkwa, O. (1999). 'Towards a national policy for the elderly in Ghana', Ageing International, vol.25, no.1, pp.31-45.

de-Graft Aikins, A. (2007). 'Ghana's neglected chronic disease epidemic: a developmental challenge', Ghana Medical Journal, vol.14, pp.154-159.

Edington, G.M. (1954). 'Cardiovascular disease as a cause of death in the Gold Coast African', Tran. Roy. Soc. Med. Hyg., vol. 48, pp. 419-425.

Gould, L, Greenland, P., Grundy,S.M., Hill, M.N., Hlatky, M.A., Houston- Miller, N., Krauss, R.M., LaRosa, J., Ockene, I.S., Oparil, S., Pearson, T.A., Rapaport, E,

Starke, R. et al. (1995). Secondary Prevention Panel . 'Preventing heart attack and death in patients with coronary disease', *Circulation,* vol.92, pp.2–4.

Hamzat, T.K. and Kobiri, A (2008). 'Effects of walking with a cane on balance and social participation among community-dwelling post-stroke individuals', Eur J Phys Rehabili Med., vol.44, no.2, pp.121-126.

Kengne, A.P and Anderson, C.S. (2006). 'The neglected burden of stroke in sub-Saharan Africa', *International Journal of Stroke,* vol.1, pp.180-190.

Moris, K. (2011). 'Collaboration works to improve stroke outcomes in Ghana', The *Lancet,* vol.377, pp.1639-1640.

Nyame, P.K., Bonsu-Bruce, N., Amoah, A.G.B., Adjei, S., Nyarko, E., Amuah, E.A. and Biritwum, R.B. (1994). 'Current Trends in the incidence of cerebrovascular accidents in Accra', *West.African.Medical Journal,* vol.13, pp.183-186.

Obajimi, M.O., Nyame, P.K., Jumah, K.B., and Wiredu, E.K. (2002), 'Spontaneous intracranial haemorrhage: computed tomographic patterns in Accra', *West Afr J Med.,* vol.21, no.2, pp.121-3.

Peltzer, K. and Pengpid, S. (2011). 'Overweight and obesity and associated factors among school-aged adolescents in Ghana and Uganda', Int. J. Environ. Res. Public Health, vol.8, pp.3859-3870.

Plange-Rhule, J., Phillips, R., Acheampong, J.W., Saggar-Malik, A.K., Cappuccio, F.P. and Eastwood, J.B. (1999). 'Hypertension and renal failurein Kumasi, Ghana', J Hum Hypertens,vol.13, no.1, pp.37-40.

Population Reference Bureau. (2012). 'World population data sheet', Washington DC,

Roberts, M.A., Opare-Sem, O.K.and Acheampong, J.W. (1994). 'The diurnal variation of stroke in Ghana', *Tropical Doctor,* vol.24, no.4, pp.155-157.

Wiredu, E.K and Nyame, P.K. (2001). 'Stroke-Related Mortality at Korle Bu Teaching Hospital Accra, Ghana', East African Medical Journal, vol. 78, pp.180–4.

World Health Organization (2012). 'Report on the top causes of deaths', WHO, Geneva, Switzerland.

Chapter 3

Diabetes in Ghana: a review of research on prevalence, experiences and healthcare

Ama de-Graft Aikins, Ellis Owusu-Dabo and Charles Agyemang

Introduction

Diabetes mellitus (also referred to as diabetes) is defined as "a chronic disease caused by inherited and/or acquired deficiency in production of insulin by the pancreas, or by the ineffectiveness of the insulin produced" (World Health Organisation, 2002. Four principal forms are distinguished (WHO, 1999). Type 1 (also known as insulin-dependent diabetes mellitus) is characterised by a failure of the pancreas to produce insulin and occurs most frequently in children and adolescents. Type 2 (also known as non-insulin-dependent diabetes mellitus) results from irregular physiological responses to insulin production and uptake, including insulin resistance at the level of the cell (and nuclear) membrane. It is attributed to lifestyle factors in adults. Gestational diabetes mellitus arises from insulin resistance and glucose intolerance during pregnancy. The final form is described as 'other specific types of diabetes' including those due to 'genetic disorders, infections, diseases of the exocrine pancreas, endocrinopathies and drugs' (Mbanya and Ramiaya, 2006: 270). Insulin deficiencies and irregularities result in increased concentrations of blood glucose, which can damage many bodily systems, but most crucially blood vessels and nerves. Left untreated, raised blood-glucose levels can lead to a range of acute and chronic medical complications. Acute complications include *ketoacidosis, hyperosmolar non-ketotic coma, hypoglycemia,* and diabetes-related infections. Chronic complications include *retinopathy, nephropathy, neuropathy* and foot complications. Other co-morbidities of diabetes include cerebrovascular events and coronary artery disease.

Diabetes is a global health problem and a major cause of morbidity, disability and death in many countries. Its effects are further heightened by the fact that it constitutes a risk factor for other serious chronic diseases such as coronary heart diseases and stroke. African countries along with poor countries of Asia and

Latin America bear a significant proportion of the global diabetes burden. Of the 177 million people living with diabetes worldwide in 2003, two-thirds lived in poor countries in Africa, Asia and Latin America (WHO, 2005). There are 10.4 million individuals with diabetes in Africa currently. It is estimated that this figure will rise by 80 percent to reach 18.7 million by 2025 (Kengne et al., 2005). If current rural-urban prevalence disparities persist, urban populations will be most affected. The burden of diabetes in Africa is also compounded by its relationship with tuberculosis and HIV/AIDS (Young et al., 2009). Current research suggests that diabetes increases the risk of TB by around threefold and thst the underlying risk is likely to be related to the impact of diabetes on the immune response and chronic inflammation. The rapidly increasing prevalence of diabetes may add to the impact of HIV infection on TB control (Unwin and Alberti, 2006). These co-morbid relationships will hit poor urban and rural communities the hardest.

Ghana has a significant diabetes burden, with a profile similar to that of other African countries (Hall et al., 2011). While diabetes, hypertension and other chronic diseases have been prioritised in official health sector documents since the early 1990s, policy recognition has not translated into concrete action (MOH, 2001, 2005, 2008; Bosu, Chapter 9, this volume). This has implications for diabetes research and interventions and on the quality of life of people living with diabetes.

In this chapter, we review research on Type 2 diabetes in Ghana since the earliest recorded prevalence study in the 1950s. We focus on three key areas where sufficient evidence exists: prevalence (to track trends in urban and rural areas); experiences (to examine everyday experiences of people living with diabetes including self-care and social support); and quality of care (to examine the facilitators and barriers to service provision for people living with diabetes). Studies on the other types of diabetes (cf. Laryea, 1978; Owusu, 1978; Kratzer, 2012), have been excluded from this review because they are too limited to for a meaningful synthesis of trends and patterns.

Methods

We conducted a standard literature review of published empirical studies on prevalence, prevention and quality of care. We searched the Pubmed and Psychinfo databases for published research on diabetes in Ghana. We hand-searched *Ghana Medical Journal* for additional research outputs on the subject.

We also accessed grey literature, including Master's and PhD theses, research reports and conference papers and proceedings. The inclusion criteria were peer-reviewed empirical studies on Type 2 diabetes, employing any method, in the three identified areas. Exclusion criteria were reviews, comment papers and other material not based on empirical research. The latter set of material provided the general context for discussion, but were not included in the synthesis of evidence reported. We identified eligible empirical studies on diabetes. The majority of studies on diabetes were conducted in the Greater Accra, Ashanti and Brong-Ahafo regions of Ghana constituting approximately 40 percent of the total population of Ghana.

Results

Prevalence of diabetes

Two kinds of diabetes prevalence studies have been conducted in Ghana. Whereas community-based studies have sought to measure diabetes prevalence in apparently healthy populations in their living or working environments, institution-based studies have been conducted in the major hospitals: Korle-Bu Teaching Hospital (Adubofour et al., 1993; Akpalu et al., 2011), Tema General Hospital (Owiredu et al., 2008; Adinortey et al., 2011) and Komfo Anokye Teaching Hospital. These are primarily observational studies which measure prevalence of diabetes and risk factors in populations of identified patients. Findings from community-based studies are highlighted in this section.

The earliest diabetes prevalence study reported was conducted in the late 1950s in a population of men in Ho in the Volta Region of Ghana. The recorded prevalence was 0.2 percent (Dodu and de Heer, 1964). In the early 1970s, Pobee and colleagues conducted a study on general and cardiovascular health among public servants in the capital city, Accra, and reported a diabetes prevalence of 0.5 percent among males and 0.4 percent among females. There are no records of further community-based studies until the early 1990s, when the Ghana Diabetes Association conducted a screening exercise in selected urban areas and reported a prevalence of around 2 percent (Bosu, 2007). In 1998, diabetes prevalence was measured in a large sample of 4,733 adult participants, aged 25 and older, from two urban communities and 20 rural communities in Accra (Amoah et al., 2002). Diabetes prevalence of 6.4 percent was reported and the rate for impaired glucose tolerance (IGT) among this sample population was 10.7 percent. A small number of prevalence studies have been conducted in the last ten years in the cities of Accra and Kumasi with prevalence rates reported ranging between 6 percent and 7 percent, while studies conducted among sedentary workers have reported higher rates. In 2003, a health survey and clinical study was conducted among 1328 adult women in Accra through a collaboration between Harvard University and the University of Ghana (Hill et al., 2007; Duda et al., 2007; Darko et al., 2012). This study, called the Accra Women's Study, reported diabetes prevalence of 8.3 percent. In 2006, Addo and colleagues (2009) reported a diabetes prevalence of 9.1 percent among 1015 civil servants in Accra and a prevalence rate of 17.4 percent for impaired fasting glucose. More recently, Amidu and colleagues (2009) conducted a study to measure the prevalence of metabolic syndrome (Mets) among a group of 100 male garage mechanics in Kumasi. They recorded a diabetes prevalence of 6.0 percent. Cook-Huynh and colleagues (2012) also conducted a study in Adankwame, a rural community approximately 12 km from Kumasi in which they report a prevalence of 8 percent among 326 adult men and women.

Although the above studies seek to shed some light on the nature and extent of diabetes in Ghana, fewer diabetes prevalence studies have been conducted than to hypertension prevalence studies (see Addo et al., Chapter 1). With the exception of the pioneering study in Ho (Dodu and de Heer, 1964), all the studies have also been concentrated in Accra and Kumasi, with none reported in other regions of the country. However, the limited evidence suggests that diabetes prevalence has increased significantly in both cities, from less than 1 percent in the 1950s through 1970s to almost 10 percent fifty years later. As Cook-Huynh and colleagues (2012) observe, the current Ghanaian rates, albeit limited to a few cities and regions of the country, are higher than the worldwide estimated prevalence of diabetes. Where studies have reported rates among men and women, prevalence rates are higher among men (Amoah et al., 2002; Addo et al., 2009; Pobee, 1991). This reflects the gender differences in diabetes prevalence in many African countries (Hall et al., 2011). Where impaired glucose tolerance and impaired fasting glucose have been measured, the rates are almost double the rates of diabetes in the target communities (Amoah et al, 2002; Addo et al., 2009). This suggests that more individuals may be at the pre-diabetes stage and may be at higher risk of developing diabetes in the future and/or that detection rates are relatively low and diabetes prevalence may be under-reported. The latter assertion is buttressed by the fact that in the community surveyed by Amoah and colleagues (2002) almost 70 percent of diabetes was undiagnosed. This finding is similar to findings in hypertension prevalence studies where high levels of undiagnosed hypertension exist (Addo et al, Chapter 1). When individuals lack awareness of their at-risk status or their cardiovascular health status, they cannot take decisions to reduce their risk and manage their health appropriately.

Diabetes experiences

The bulk of evidence on diabetes experiences comes from a series of published studies based on a large-scale qualitative study of diabetes conducted between 2000 and 2001 in Accra, and Tema in the Greater Accra Region and Nkoranza and Kintampo in the Brong-Ahafo Region (de-Graft Aikins, 2003, 2004, 2005, 2006). More recently an anthropological study of serious sickness (including diabetes) among Ga communities in Accra has been conducted, and some findings have been published (Atobrah, 2012). Medical studies, which have employed questionnaires and scales to examine patient knowledge of diabetes and aspects of self-care and complications, also provide some relevant insights (Ofei et al., 2002; Owiredu et al., 2011).

To understand experiences it is important to understand how individuals with diabetes conceptualise causes and implications of diabetes and available resources for diabetes management. The reported qualitative studies suggest that diabetes is attributed to a range of interchangeable causes: high sugar diets, heredity, physiological imbalance, toxic foods and supernatural causes (witchcraft, sorcery). High sugar diets and physiological imbalance are deemed primary causes, for which biomedicine offers the most successful solutions. The level of sophistication of biomedical explanations of diabetes increases with education, however both uneducated and educated participants hold sufficient biomedical knowledge on diabetes to prioritize drug treatment and diet management over alternative medical and self-care practices.

People living with diabetes experience psychosocial challenges. The psychosocial impact of chronic disease straddles the psychological-social continuum of everyday experiences of chronic illness. This continuum encompasses at one end the emotional and psychological responses to the physical and life-changing impact of long-term illness and at the other end the structural impact of living with a long-term condition such as healthcare access and costs. In between, individuals deal with the social and cultural implications of illness, such as the way socio-cultural representations of the illness and responses to the individual with the illness strengthen or undermine social support.

The general literature on diabetes reports strong associations between diabetes experiences and emotional and psychological distress, in particular depression (Leone et al., 2012). The local research reports similar associations. The studies by de-Graft Aikins (2003, 2004, 2005, 2006) examine the psychosocial impact of diabetes through the concept of 'biographical disruption'. Coined by the medical sociologist Michael Bury (1982), biographical disruption refers to the way chronic disease disrupts the physical body and the life trajectory of individuals living with the disease, and the responses evoked by the disruption. Diabetes causes physical problems and complications, ranging from the minor (general tiredness) to the major (sexual dysfunction, blindness). Individuals have to deal with the physical impairments and disabilities that come with the condition or its complications.

Diabetes also disrupts social identities and social roles. When individuals lose a limb, or their eyesight fails, the disability changes their identities, in their own eyes and in the eyes of their significant others. Men who experience sexual dysfunction (see for example Owiredu et al., 2012) through the side effects of diabetes medications or through diabetes complications struggle to manage their lost or diminished masculine identities. Disrupted social identities do not come only from the physical impairments or disabilities, but also from the implications these pose for individuals' ability to work and earn a living. For example, some farmers in Kintampo and Nkoranza have to abandon their farming or develop new strategies, such as hiring farm help, to maintain their primary occupation.

Beyond the emotional and psychological impact, diabetes has a financial impact. The WHO (2005) has observed that chronic diseases push individuals and families into poverty and poverty undermines health outcomes for individuals living with chronic diseases. Treating diabetes in Ghana is expensive for both low- and high-income people. Low-income individuals struggle to cover medical costs as well as costs for everyday management of diabetes such as prescribed healthy diets. The high cost of care has a major influence on the healthcare choices individuals made.

Finally, the quality of social relationships changes within the context of chronic conditions. The changes range from a switch in social roles in the home to experiences of enhanced or dwindling social support. Ghanaians with diabetes rely largely on a restricted set of family members for social and financial support. In poor areas of Accra, Kintampo and Nkoranza, social and financial support is variable and not guaranteed to be long term, due to the financial insecurities of broader family systems. In rural areas and provincial towns such as Kintampo and Nkoranza, individuals living with uncontrolled diabetes and associated rapid sustained weight loss experience HIV/AIDS-related stigma (de-Graft Aikins, 2006). Their caregivers also experience stigma by association; what the sociologist Erving Goffman (1963) has referred to as 'courtesy stigma'. There is a greater tendency for women with diabetes in Nkoranza to be divorced or abandoned by their partners or stigmatised by their communities. The gendered nature of diabetes experiences works in the opposite direction, especially in the area of identity management among men with sexual health problems arising from diabetes treatment and complications.

Ghana, like many African countries, has a vibrant and dynamic pluralistic medical system. In addition to biomedical services, ethnomedical services, faith healers (belonging to evangelical Christian churches or independent African churches) and non-African complementary therapies (e.g. Chinese, Ayurveda, etc) exist and offer care for a variety of diseases. Diabetes is on the list of diseases.

People with diabetes shop for healing within and across these systems. Healer-shopping, a term derived from doctor-shopping, has been defined as "the use of a second healer without referral from the first for a single episode of illness" (Kroeger, 1983: 147, cited by de-Graft Aikins, 2005). Healer-shopping has been attributed to the high cost of biomedical care, coupled with the psychosocial burden of diabetes which sets the majority of individuals on a course of either passive or active cure-seeking (de-Graft Aikins, 2005). Different choices (within or across systems) depend on individuals' socio-economic status and access to these pluralistic services, as well as on whether individuals hope for a biomedical breakthrough, or believe in a (Christian) spiritual cure for diabetes (ibid).

Knowledge of these pluralistic services is drawn from a variety of sources: lifeworlds (of family, friends and social networks;) mass media (including adverts placed by various medical practitioners), social and religious spaces (e.g. churches, mosques, social organisations such as lodges, Rotary clubs etc), and engagement with the systems themselves (e.g. within and across system referrals).

Individuals and communities are reported to evaluate biomedicine, ethnomedicine and faith-healing systems along four criteria: technical or practical knowledge of health problems, technological expertise, (geographic, economic, cultural) accessibility, and ethics. All systems have strengths and weaknesses across these criteria, depending on the health problem.

Biomedicine is preferred for its diagnostic and treatment expertise. It is important to note that prioritization of biomedical care over other forms of care does not necessarily imply exclusive use of biomedical services. In a study examining the structure and processes of healer-shopping, de-Graft Aikins (2005) reported that participants who remained committed to biomedical management belonged to a group with three distinct or interlinked experiences: (1) individuals who had lived with diabetes long term; (2) individuals who had experienced few or no life disruptions from diabetes; and (3) individuals who lived with other serious conditions, such as hypertension and prostate cancer. For this group, practical daily routines were geared towards controlling symptoms through drug and diet management, and routine lifestyle change (drinking less, taking up exercise).

Of the three systems, faith healers pose the greatest risks to people with diabetes. Their method of treatment is usually prayer and fasting or 'deliverance': fasting as a primary healing strategy has been known to place diabetes sufferers at risk of hypoglycaemia.

Diabetes care

In the mid-1990s, a major project was conducted to examine the burden of diabetes and medical and lay responses to the condition. This project, referred to in local medical circles as the Ghana Diabetes Project, was a collaboration between the two medical schools (University of Ghana Medical School and Kwame Nkrumah University of Science and Technology) and the University of Virgina, US. The project was funded by the US drug company Eli Lilly. The Ghana Diabetes Project was the first major attempt to examine the capacity of major hospitals to respond to the growing burden of diabetes in the country. The project researchers reported the following:

"Ghana has no diabetes advisory board and no guidelines for diabetes care for the various healthcare levels. Diabetic medications are not tax-exempt. Diabetes registers are available for only the two teaching hospitals. No data are available on diabetes mortality, morbidity and disability. A general deficiency in facilities and resources for diabetes care exists in health facilities and there is an erratic supply of essential diabetes products at health institutions. Diabetes care in Ghana has hitherto been largely uncoordinated with no formal national policy on diabetes. This is in spite of the 2006 UN declaration on diabetes calling on all governments "to develop national policies for prevention, treatment and care of diabetes in line with the sustainable development of their health care systems" (IDF, 2010). In 2010, the International Diabetes Fderation (IDF) published a comprehensive guideline for national diabetes programmes which if adopted and adapted within the context of Ghana would make a significant impact on current diabetes practice. Major hindrances to current diabetes care and practice in Ghana include lack of trained diabetes health care personnel and lack of the team approach to diabetes care" (Amoah et al., 2000: 150).

The earlier observations made in 2000 still hold true for diabetes care in Ghana 13 years later. In terms of the health care system or infrastructure, Ghana has 10 regional hospitals, 65 district hospitals, 400 health centres and about 1200 service delivery points referred to as CHPS zones. However there are only two specialist diabetes centres in the country: the diabetes centres at Korle Bu Teaching Hospital in the capital Accra and Komfo Anokye Teaching Hospital in the Ashanti regional capital, Kumasi. Both centres are located in, and serve the urban south, which means people living with diabetes in the rural south and north face rising levels of difficulty in accessing specialist diabetes care. The regional hospitals across the country treat diabetes through regular clinics, but they lack specialists. Poor public and patient knowledge has been associated, in part, with poor communication practices by public health and biomedical professionals. Technical terms usually in English are widely used in communication strategies. These do not translate easily for the lay public, both uneducated and educated. Nutrition and dietetics, in particular, are underdeveloped in diabetes care across the country. Gatiba and colleagues (2007) demonstrate that while lack of education or poor education undermines nutrition knowledge, poor nutrition knowledge can also be attributed to dieticians' use of linguistically unfamiliar nutritional terms such as 'minerals, proteins and vitamins'. The lack of specialist diabetes care is symptomatic of a general lack of specialist care for chronic diseases in Ghana, and much of sub-Saharan Africa (Mensah, 2008; Hall et al., 2011; de-Graft Aikins et al., 2010).

The medical cost of diabetes care is high for all income groups. However, poor individuals in rural and urban areas experience chronic financial insecurities due to diabetes (de-Graft Aikins, 2005). The National Health Insurance Scheme (NHIS) was established in 2006 and some diabetes medicines were placed on the exemption list. This has eased the financial cost of diabetes care for some individuals. However, access to NHIS requires payment of the annual premium which may be too expensive for the poorest individuals, especially in rural communities. Secondly, the scheme is facing teething problems, such as delays in reimbursing hospitals for cost of medications, which impacts on drug procurement, which has significant implications on continuity of care for long-term chronic conditions. It is important to factor in other costs of care such as travel, waiting time at health centres and diet management. These tend to affect the rural and urban poor with diabetes disproportionately.

Healer-shopping, as noted earlier, is a key feature of healthcare choices people with diabetes make. Experts perceive healershopping negatively, and link complications and premature deaths to patients' engagement with harmful diagnostic and treatment practices of alternative medical systems. Researchers working on plant medicine suggest that ethnopharmaceutical medicines exist and may offer affordable and clinically effective alternatives to people living with a variety of chronic conditions, including diabetes. A unique service is provided by the Centre for Scientific Research into Plant Medicine (CSRPM), a centre that offers biomedical care with a mix of standard pharmaceutical drugs and pharmacologically and clinically tested 'ethnopharmaceuticals'. The centre is based in Aburi in the Eastern Region (less than thirty minutes drive from the outskirts of Accra) and serves clients, including people with diabetes, from the Eastern region and neighbouring regions of Greater Accra and Ashanti. People with diabetes who use the services of CSRPM rate the services positively. However, the cost of travel can be high and can undermine continuous engagement in care (de-Graft Aikins, 2005).

Social support is crucial to self-care and coping. In Ghana, family members often bear sole responsibility for social support, as discussed previously. However, over the last ten years, diabetes self-help groups have emerged in a number of regions, including Greater Accra, Ashanti, Brong Ahafo and Upper East. Most groups are usually set up by doctors or senior nurses and co-run by the founders and patients on a voluntary basis. More recently, peer support groups have been set up by people living with diabetes (A. Aifah, personal communication, July, 2011). All patient and support groups focus on basic diabetes education and some psychosocial support. The Ghana Diabetes Association (GDA), the national body representing people with diabetes, is based in Accra and often limits its (primarily advocacy) activities to Accra or the southern towns. The GDA is supposed to have regional branches but these are not as active as the national umbrella organisation. The smaller community-based self-help groups do not appear to be linked formally to GDA (A. Aifah, personal communication, July, 2011).

Conclusions

The prevalence of diabetes has increased over time, from less than 1 percent in the late 1950s to 1970s in rural and urban areas to almost 10 percent in urban areas in 2009. The condition affects both urban and rural populations. Adult men appear to have a higher risk of diabetes than adult women. People living with diabetes are reported to have sufficient biomedical knowledge of the condition to set ideal self-care goals. However, the complex everyday experience of diabetes undermines good self-care intentions. People with diabetes live with psychological and emotional difficulties (anxiety, depression) linked to the complex burden of living with diabetes, including the daily difficulties of complying with drug and diet management and dealing with minor and major physical impairments, the financial cost of treatment, reduction in physical capabilities and negative social responses to their changed identities. Despite policy attention to diabetes in the early 1990s (see Bosu, Chapter 9) there has been minimal improvement in diabetes care. There are few diabetes specialists and knowledge of diabetes among health professionals is poor. This affects the quality of diabetes care. Compared to hypertension research (see Addo et al., Chapter 1), diabetes research is limited and has been concentrated in Accra and Kumasi. More information is needed on trends in diabetes prevalence across the country and on the rural-urban and gender differences.

It will be useful for future studies to include measures of risk factors like obesity, cholesterol levels, dietary practice, smoking and alcohol use. Similarly, studies on lay knowledge and experiences of diabetes are limited. To develop better diabetes education interventions and quality patient-centred care, it is important to understand community representations of diabetes as well as responses to diabetes, both in terms of people living with the condition and those providing care for sufferers. Two new projects have been initiated that aim to examine these aspects of diabetes. One project, a New York University-funded collaboration with the University of Ghana, led locally by the University of Ghana Medical School, aims to develop and analyse a database of diabetic patients attending the diabetes clinic at the Korle-Bu Teaching Hospital. The second project, led locally by the Regional Institute for Population Studies and the School of Public Health, aims to develop a task-shifting approach to hypertension and diabetes care in Accra. The RODAM – Risk of Obesity and Diabetes among African Migrants - project is a collaborative project between the University of Amsterdam, London School of Hygiene and Tropical Medicine, Charité – University Medicine, Berlin, German Institute for Nutrition Research, The International Diabetes Federation, Africa Region;, Kwame Nkrumah University of Science and Technology; and the University of Ghana. Funded by the European Union, the RODAM project aims to examine the risk of obesity and diabetes among Ghanaian migrants in the United Kingdom, Netherlands and Germany and their compatriots at home, in rural and urban Ashanti Region. The project involves quantitative measures, qualitative measures and objective measures on blood pressure, blood glucose and related biomarkers. Although these new projects are based in Accra and Kumasi, they mark a significant departure from previous diabetes studies in three ways. They are multi-disciplinary in conceptualisation and methods. They incorporate postgraduate diabetes research training in the medical and social sciences. They aim to offer a new wave of comprehensive data from a new set of affected communities that facilitates nuanced analysis of the interplay between the medical, psychological, social and structural dimensions of diabetes.

References

Addo J, Smeeth L, Leon DA (2009) Hypertensive Target Organ Damage in Ghanaian Civil Servants with Hypertension. PLoS ONE 4(8): e6672. doi:10.1371/journal.pone.0006672

Adinortey, M.B., Gyan, B.E., Adjimani, J., Nyarko, P., Sarpong, C., Francis Y. Tsikata, F.Y. and Nyarko, A.K (2011). Dyslipidaemia Associated with Type 2 Diabetics with Micro and Macrovascular Complications among Ghanaians. *Indian Journal of Clinical Biochemistry*, 26(3):261–268

Adubofuor, K.O.M., Ofei, F., Mensah-Adubofour, J., Owusu, S.K. (1993). Diabetes in Ghana: a morbidity and mortality analysis. *International Diabetes Digest*. 4(3), 90-92.

Adubofou,r K.O.M., Ofei, F., Mensah-Adubufour J, Owusu S.K. (1997). Diabetes in Ghana. In Gill G, Mbanya J-C, Alberti G (Eds), *Diabetes in Africa*. Eds. Gill G, Mbanya J-C, Alberti G . FSG Communications Ltd, Reach, Cambridge, UK. (pp. 83-88)

Amidu, N., Owiredu, W.K.B.A., Mireku, E.K and Agyemang, C. (2012). Metabolic syndrome among garage workers in the automobile industry in Kumasi, Ghana. *Journal of Medical* and Biomedical Sciences, 1(3): 29-36

Amoah A.G, Owusu, S.K., Saunders, J.T., Fang, W.L., Asare, H.A., Pastors, J.G, Sanborn, C, Barrett, E.J., Woode, M.K., Osei. K. (1998). Facilities and resources for diabetes care at regional health facilities in southern Ghana. *Diabetes Res Clin Pract*. 42(2):123-30.

Amoah, A.G.B, Owusu, S.K., Acheampong, J.W., Agyenim-Boateng K., Asare, H.R, Owusu, A.A., Mensah-Poku, M.F., Adamu F.C., Amegashie, R.A., Saunders, J.T, Fang, W.L., Pastors, J.G.,Sanborn, C., Barrett, E.J., and Woode, M.K (2000). A national diabetes care and education programme: the Ghana model. *Diabetes Research and Clinical Practice*, 49(2-3):149-57.

Amoah, A.G.B, Owusu, K.O., and Adjei, S (2002). Diabetes in Ghana: a community prevalence study in Greater Accra. *Diabetes Research and Clinical Practice*, 56: 197-205.

Amoah, A.G.B. (2002). Undiagnosed diabetes and impaired glucose regulation in adult Ghanaians using the ADA and WHO diagnostic criteria. *Acta Diabetol*, 39(1), 7-13.

Cook-Huynh, M., Ansong, D., Steckelberg, R.C., Boakye, I., Seligman, K., Appiah, L., Kumar, N., Amuasi, J.H. (2012). Prevalence of hypertension and diabetes mellitus in adults from a rural community in Ghana. *Ethnicity and Disease*, 22(3):347–352.

Darko, R., Adanu, R.M., Duda, R.B., Douptcheva, N., Hill, A.G. (2012). The health of adult women in Accra, Ghana: self-reporting and objective assessments 2008-2009. *Ghana Medical Journal*, 46:2.

de-Graft Aikins, A. (2002). Exploring biomedical and ethnomedical representations of diabetes in Ghana and the scope for cross-professional collaboration: a social psychological approach to health policy. *Social Science Information*, 41(4), 603-630.

de-Graft Aikins, A (2003). Living with diabetes in rural and urban Ghana: a critical social psychological examination of illness action and scope for intervention. *Journal of Health Psychology*, 8(5),557-72.

de-Graft Aikins, A (2004). Strengthening quality and continuity of diabetes care in rural Ghana: a critical social psychological approach. *Journal of Health Psychology*, 2004, 9(2), 295-309.

de-Graft Aikins, A (2005). Healer-shopping in Africa: new evidence from a rural-urban qualitative study of Ghanaian diabetes experiences. *British Medical Journal*, 331, 737.

de-Graft Aikins, A. (2006) Reframing applied disease stigma research: a multilevel analysis of diabetes stigma in Ghana. *Journal of Community and Applied Social Psychology*, 16(6), 426-441.

de-Graft Aikins, A., Unwin, N., Agyemang, C. Allotey, P., Campbell, C and Arhinful, D.K (2010). Editoral:Africa's Chronic Disease Burden: local and global perspectives. *Globalization and Health*, 5/6.

de-Graft Aikins, A., Anum, A., Agyemang, C., Addo, J. and Ogedegbe, O.(2012). Lay representations of chronic diseases in Ghana: implications for primary prevention. Ghana Medical Journal, 46(2), 59-68.

Dodu, S.R.A and de Heer, N. (1964).A diabetes case-finding survey in Ho. *Ghana Medical* Journal, 1964; 3:75-80.

Duda, R.B., Darko, R., Seffah, J., Adanu, R.M.K., Anarfi, J.K.,Allan G. Hill, A.G. (2007). Prevalence of Obesity in Women of Accra, Ghana.*African Journal of Health Science, 14, 154-159.*

Goffman, E. (1963/1990). Stigma: Notes on the management of spoiled identity. New Jersey: Prentice-Hall.

Hall, V., Thomsen, R.W., Henriksen, O., Lohse, N. (2011).Diabetes in Sub Saharan Africa 1999-2011: Epidemiology and public health implications. A systematic review. BMC Public Health 2011, 11:564

Hill, A.G., Darko, R., Seffah, J., Adanu, R.M., Anarfi, J.K., Duda, R.B. (2007). Health of urban Ghanaian women as identified by the Women's Health Study of Accra. Int J Gynaecol Obstet;99(2):150–156.

Laryea, E. A. (1978), Diabetes mellitus complicating pregnancy, *Ghana Medical Journal*, Vol.17, 224-228.

Leone, T., Coast, E., Narayanan, S and de-Graft Aikins, A.(2012) Diabetes and depression comorbidity within poor settings in low and middle income countries (LMICs): a mapping of the evidence. *Globalization and Health*, 8:39.

Mensah GA: Epidemiology of stroke and high blood pressure in Africa. *Heart* 2008, 94:697-705.

Monitoring and Evaluation Team (1998). Formative and Baseline Research on Diabetes Mellitus in Ghana. Ghana Diabetes Care and Disease Management Project.Eli Lilly & Co. Monitoring and Evaluation Team (2001). Evaluation of a 3-Year Training Programme in Diabetes Mellitus for Health Care Professionals. Ghana Diabetes Care and Disease Management Project.Eli Lilly & Co.

Noordermeer, C. (2007). Diabetes care in Ghana: an exploratory study in Greater Accra Region. 2007, Unpublished MSc Thesis, 2007,Vrije Universiteit Amsterdam.

Ofei F, Forson A, and Appia-Kusi J. (2002). A preliminary study of self-care behaviour among Ghanaians with diabetes mellitus.*Ghana Medical Journal*, 36(ii):54-59

Owiredu, W.K.B.A., Amidu, N, Alidu, H., Sarpong, C., and Gyasi-Sarpong, C.K. (2011). Determinants of sexual dysfunction among clinically diagnosed diabetic patients. *Reproductive Biology and Endocrinology* 2011, 9:70

Rotimi C, Daniel H, Zhou J, Obisesan A, Chen G, Chen Y, Amoah A, Opoku V, Acheampong J, Agyenim-Boateng K, Eghan, B.A. Jr, Oli J, Okafor G, Ofoegbu E, Osotimehin B, Abbiyesuku F, Johnson T, Fasanmade O, Doumatey A, Aje T, Collins F, Dunston G. (2003).Prevalence and determinants of diabetic retinopathy and cataracts in West African type 2 diabetes patients. *Ethn and Disease*, 13(2 Suppl 2):S110-7.

Chapter 4.

Breast cancer research in Ghana: a focus on social science perspectives

Deborah Atobrah

Introduction

Cancers are a major cause of morbidity and mortality worldwide (GLOBOCAN, 2004). They are one of the most dreaded chronic diseases, usually resulting in intense debilitation of the human body, high cost of treatment, and massive psychological and social burden on patients, their family and social networks. There are over 150 types of cancer and each type varies in etiology, risk factors, treatment and management (O'Toole. 2003).

Scholarly attention given to cancers in developing countries is scanty, as compared to developed countries. This situation is disturbing in the light of the overwhelmingly increasing rates of detection and reporting of cancer and other non-communicable diseases in developing countries including Ghana (Parkin et a., 2004; de Graft Aikins et al., 2010). While certain cancers are curable when detected early, in Ghana, the disease is associated with low survival rates because of late presentation and detection. This further deepens feelings of fear and uncertainty on those diagnosed and their associates (Quartey-Papafio, 1977, 1980; Clegg-Lamptey et al., 2009; Opoku et al., 2012; Mayo and Hunter, 2003).

Biomedical interventions include surgery, radiotherapy, chemotherapy, immunotherapy, hormone therapy and other drug treatments (O'Toole, 2003). Furthermore, there are highly differentiated trajectories of the various cancers from the first symptom through treatment and prognosis, all of which present significant socio-cultural, economic and religious challenges to individuals and their families. In this respect, in many societies, cancer evokes a wide range of complex reactions including myths, misperceptions and problematic beliefs (Helman, 1981; Kubler-Ross, 1969). The role of social science research in understanding cancer epidemiology, the social dynamics, impact and their implications for management within a socio-cultural context cannot be overlooked. In many industrialized countries the precarious effects of neglecting social science and behavioural research in cancer discourse has long been acknowledged (Marrow et al., 1994). Auxiliary care in psychosocial, physical, practical, spiritual/existential and finance are also becoming very important in enhancing the quality of life of patients, their family and close associates who are directly and indirectly affected by the disease.

This chapter aims to provide an overview of the current state of cancer research in Ghana, with specific reference to social science perspectives on breast cancer. The lack of social science research is discussed and further areas of critical social science research recommended.

Methods

A literature search was conducted of all journal articles on cancer-related research conducted in Ghana. The author, with the assistance of two national service personnel at the Institute of African Studies (Charity Akpably and Andrew Quarty) conducted an online search through the Google Scholar search engine, with the key words *cancer* and *Ghana*. Electronic and manual searches of published articles in the *Ghana Medical Journal* were also utilized for the study. The search identified 105 journal articles published on cancer related topics in Ghana between 1956 and 2012. Two articles were not accessible. Therefore, 103 were reviewed for this chapter.

General Overview of Cancer Studies in Ghana

While there are over 150 types of cancers identified by biomedical practitioners (O'Toole, 2003), journal publications on cancer in Ghana focused only on 21 specific types of cancers as illustrated in Table 4.1 below. Breast cancer, being the commonest female cancer worldwide has been written on most, accounting for 32.4 percent of the articles published. Cervical cancer ranked second in publications frequency. Although the latter is curable when detected early through screening, it remains the second commonest cancer in many developing countries including Ghana. Eighty percent of global cervical cancer cases occur in developing countries (Ferlay et al., 2008). Nearly a third (n=14) of cervical cancer publications and half of the publications on Burkitt's Lymphoma (n=6) were based on outputs from large scale research projects. Consistent with worldwide trends, prostate cancer is the commonest male cancer in Ghana (Ferlay et al., 2008), but appears to have received little attention, with a research and publication frequency of five (5). Many of the other cancers (e.g. orofacial, laryngeal, head and neck, vulva, liver, anus) have publication frequencies between 3 and 1 (Table 4.1). The current paucity of research information on these cancers is lamentable. However the available evidence provides important insights and the basis to develop extensive and robust research on cancers in Ghana.

Table 4.1: Frequency of Publications on Cancer in Ghana by Cancer Type

	Type of Cancer	Frequency	Percentages
1	Breast	34	32.4
2	Cervical	14	13.3
3	Burkitt's Lymphoma	12	11.4
4	General Cancers	6	5.7
5	Prostate	6	5.7
6	Colorectum	5	4.8
7	Nasopharyngeal	3	2.9
8	Orofacial	3	2.9
9	Head And Neck	3	2.9
10	Breast And Cervical	2	1.9
11	Larynx	2	1.9
12	Pancreas	2	1.9
13	Skin-Related	2	1.9
14	Salivary Gland	2	1.9
15	Retinoblastoma	1	1.0
16	Neutropenia	1	1.0
17	Genitourinary	1	1.0
18	Vulva	1	1.0
19	Liver	1	1.0
20	Anus	1	1.0
21	Gynaecological	1	1.0
22	Unavailable	2	1.9
	Total	105	100

Table 4.2 presents data on the cancer literature by type of publication, main methodological approach, research/academic discipline, site of study, and sample selection. Of the 103 publications reviewed, 89.5 percent (n=94) were based on empirical research, 86.7 percent (n=91) were conducted using a quantitative approach, 86.7 percent (n=91) were biomedical in nature with

about 57.1 percent (n=60) of the studies conducted in either the Korle-Bu Teaching Hospital (KBTH) or Komfo Anokye Teaching Hospital (KATH), or jointly at both teaching hospitals. Overall, 78.1 percent (n=82) of the studies were conducted in a health facility and thus involved patient data. Eighty-five percent (n=89) of reports were based on retrospective studies relying on hospital records and not involving live participants.

Table 4.2: Profile of Cancer Publications in Ghana

VARIABLES	FREQUENCY (f)	PERCENTAGE VALUES (%)
Type of Publication		
Case Reports	6	5.7
Research	94	89.5
Systematic Reviews	3	2.9
Type of Research Conducted		
Qualitative	11	10.5
Quantitative	91	86.7
Triangulation	1	1.0
Discipline of Study		
Biomedical	94	89.5
Social Science	5	4.8
Multi/ interdisciplinary	4	3.8
Site of Study		
Korle Bu Hospital	50	47.6
Komfo Anokye Hospital	10	9.5
Multi site	30	28.6
Accra	2	1.9
Kumasi	3	2.9
Unclassified	7	6.7
Obuasi	1	1.0
Sample Selection		
Retrospective	89	84.8
Live Participants	14	13.3
Hospital Study	82	78.1
Community-based Study	21	20.0
Study conducted as part of a large-scale project[1]	24	22.9
Non-large scale project	79	75.2

1   Examples of large scale projects are the Burkitt's Tumor Project in Ghana established in 1965, and the Women Health Study of Accra conducted in 2003, both of which generated several articles on Burkitt's Tumor and cervical cancer respectively.

Breast cancer

Breast cancer is the single most studied cancer in Ghana, comprising about 32.4 percent of all published studies. Out of the 34 journal articles on breast cancer reviewed, 28 were purely biomedical studies, 6 in the social sciences. Virtually all the biomedical studies were conducted using hospital retrospective data, with the KBTH and the KATH being the two main sites for these studies. There were only two qualitative studies conducted in communities (Mayo and Hunter, 2003). It is worth noting that the KBTH and KATH until recently were the two major specialist referral hospitals in Ghana and would therefore receive the majority of cases requiring specialist interventions including breast cancer treatment. However, the fact that published research is based mainly on data from these two hospitals would therefore suggest the possibility of under-reporting of these conditions throughout the country. The true national prevalence of breast cancer may therefore not be known and any attempts to generalize on breast cancer pathology nationally using such reported figures must therefore be taken with a degree of caution.

Early studies on breast cancer in Ghana, published in the late 1970s focused on providing preliminary insights into the disease. One of the first studies that analyzed the main types of breast diseases at the KBTH between 1968 and 1971 established that "cancer of the breast, predominantly a female disease, is not rare at Korle Bu"(Aidoo, 1973). Other studies focused on disease prevalence (Aidoo,, 1973), diagnosis and treatment (Quartey-Papafio, 1977 and 1978), and pathological analyses of surgical material (Anim, 1979). Within this period, knowledge of the disease was limited, all the studies were conducted at the KBTH, and new cases of breast cancer recorded in the hospital were significantly low, totaling 176 between 1971 and 1975 (Quartey-Papafio 1977).

Over the years since, studies on cancer of the breast have included an examination of the nature of the disease, reviewing surgical material of lumps (Anim, 1979, Ohene Yeboah, 2005), and the clinicopathological features of female breast cancer (Quartey-Papafio, 1978; Agyei-Frimpong et al., 2008; Bewtra, 2010). Studies on biomedical treatment and survival are important in proving insights into treatment options, their relative efficacy in relation to recovery, survival and mortality rates (Baako and Badoe, 2001; Quartey-Papafio, 1977; Clegg-Lamptey et al., 2007). Biomedical studies on the risks, presentation, diagnosis, pattern and profile of the disease have also featured prominently in breast cancer research in Ghana (Boyle, 2012; Clegg-Lamptey et al., 2007; Ohene Yeboah and Adjei, 2012; Stark et al., 2010; Asumanu et al., 2000; Quartey-Papafio, 1977, 1978; Clegg-Lamptey et al., 2009; Aidoo, 1973; Pieris et al., 2012).

Male breast cancers have also attracted the interest of biomedical researchers. The focus of research has been the pathological characteristics of male breast cancer (Akosa et al., 2005). Male breast cancer is rare worldwide, accounting for about 1 percent of all breast cancers. Prevalence has however been reported to be higher among Black Africans, about 2.4 percent (Akosa et al., 1999) requiring more research attention and focus to establish the etiological factors and its national history in the male population.

Although the early studies on breast cancer conducted in the late 1960s and the 1970s were biomedical, there was a strong awareness of the impact of social factors on disease diagnosis, treatment and management. Patients' late presentation at a health facility was attributed to supernatural beliefs, suspicions, taboos, and lack of knowledge (Quartey-Papafio, 1977). Late presentation is problematic because it leads to late detection, unfavourable treatment outcomes, poor prognosis, and poor health service utilization (Clegg-Lamptey, 2009a). This combination of social factors has potential consequences on treatment and prognosis which is borne out by the fact that although breast cancer incidence rates are lower for African women, mortality rates are much higher and late presentation has been identified as a contributory factor (Stark et al., 2010, Clegg- Lamptey 2009a).

One would have expected that decades down the line, increased awareness and public education on breast cancer would have changed attitudes but this does not appear to be the case. Clegg-Lamptey and Hodasi (2007) report that 60 percent-70 percent patients continue to report at an advance stage of the disease, and many others abscond during treatment as a result of previous medical consultation, ignorance, fear of mastectomy, financial incapability, herbal treatment and attendance at prayers/prayer camps.

The socio-cultural context of breast cancer: insights from social science research

The dominant social science questions raised by biomedical researchers have centered on late presentation and discontinuation of biomedical treatment i.e. patient non-compliance to treatment. The few studies which have focused on social science research on breast cancer (6 out 34) have provided some useful insights into breast cancer in Ghana. The strength of these studies lie in their provision of insights into patients' attitudes and behaviour, as well as indications for future research as discussed below. These discussions fall under four main interrelated themes: psychosocial; socio cultural; religious and economic.

The psychosocial aspects of cancer experiences

The effects of psychosocial factors on patients' beliefs, attitudes and behaviour towards breast cancer dominate the scanty social science literature. In a study of 109 women in Ghana on their fatalistic beliefs on breast cancer, Mayo and Hunter (2003) discovered a communication challenge whereby respondents were reluctant to mention the name "cancer" for fear of attracting the disease. This is consistent with the study of Field (1961) and Atobrah (2009), indicating how abstaining from mentioning the name of a chronic disease is perceived as a traditional mode of disease prevention among the Ga of Accra. Intense fear is then exhibited when patients experience any symptoms and see signs of the disease. The study of Clegg-Lamptey et al., (2009b) which explored why patients report late or abscond from treatment corroborates this assertion (Clegg-Lamptey et al., 2009a). In their study, they found that out of 14 reasons given by patients for reporting late at the KBTH, fear of mastectomy ranked 3rd and fear of diagnosis ranked 7th. In total, 55 of the 66 patients in their study studied admitted various kinds of fear including fear of death. Fear of mastectomy was the primary reason why patients absconded from treatment. In another observational study focusing on the psychosocial aspects of breast cancer treatments, by Clegg-Lamptey et al., (2009a), fear featured prominently as a psychosocial challenge for patients in respect of death and mastectomy/deformity. Cost of treatment, uncertain future, job and marriage security, stigmatization, hospitalization, alopecia, and pain were other expressions of fear among patients. Only 8 out of the 89 patients interviewed in the later study did not express such fears (Clegg-Lamptey et al.,, 2009a). In this study, nearly 61 percent of respondent experienced psychosocial challenges because they lacked the opportunity to communicate their fear of death. In a qualitative study comparing the experiences of breast cancer and AIDS patients on stigmatization, Antwi and Atobrah, (2006) did not find breast cancer patients to have experienced much stigmatization. Patients' fear in this regard is therefore one of perceived stigma rather than actual stigma. Although Opoku et al., (2012) also discovered that fear of death tops attitudes of 474 respondents, a sense of guilt also featured strongly in the range of psychosocial reactions experienced by breast cancer patients.

Generally, patients' fears may be warranted in view of the common knowledge of the apparent poor prognosis of most cancers worldwide. Kubler-Ross, (1969) describes in five discrete states the process by which people deal with grief and tragedy especially when diagnosed with a terminal disease: denial, anger, bargaining, depression and acceptance. Adopting Kubler-Ross's model of the stages of grief, Atobrah, (2012) analyses how young patients diagnosed with cancer or other chronic diseases experience prolonged periods of denial as a result of fear. This was noted to influence their help-seeking and health-seeking behaviours by living as though there was nothing wrong with them.

The socio-cultural aspects of cancer experiences

Fear and psychosocial reactions of breast cancer patients (including shock and depression) as noted by Clegg-Lamptey et al., (2009a) also have their roots in socio-cultural norms, beliefs and expectations of the 'breast cancer experience'. Drawing on an ethnographic study of the Ga people, Atobrah, (2009) has illustrated how traditional notions of disease causality and culture-appropriate disease treatment influence patients' health and help-seeking behaviour. Breast cancer being mainly a female disease is also very likely to be influenced by socio-cultural gender norms and practices as mentioned by Opoku et al., (2012). The frequent usage of, and reliance on herbal and traditional medicines by individuals living with cancer (Clegg-Lamptey et al. 2009a, 2009b; Opoku et al, 2012) reflects the general health-seeking practices of many Ghanaians (Twumasi, 1975, Tsey 1997). Socio-cultural practices however ought not to be always seen as obstructive to biomedical treatments of breast cancer. In the absence of hospices for palliative care, the extended family system has provided ample non-medical care and support for most patients, particularly at the terminal stages of the condition (Atobrah, 2009).

The economic aspects of cancer experiences

Cancer prevention, management and control impose high financial burdens at the governmental, ministerial, institutional and individual levels. A recent study by Zelle and colleagues (2012) seems to be the only study which analyses costs and financial aspects of breast cancer in Ghana. The authors examine costs, effects and cost-effectiveness of breast cancer control in Ghana. They indicate biennial screening by clinical breast examination (CBE) as the most cost-effective intervention for women aged 40-49 years in combination with treatment of all stages, costing $1,299 per DALY. Mass media awareness -raising and mammography screening were the second and third most cost-effective options respectively. The socio-economic burden on breast cancer patients and their families is huge and although no studies focusing on this theme were noted, the issues emerged in some of the literature. At the individual level, patients' financial incapability was listed as an important reason why many breast cancer patients abscond and discontinue the very essential medical treatment (Clegg-Lamptey, 2009). The medical regimens for diagnosing and treating cancers are demanding and have huge financial implications. Patients are usually required to have several laboratory investigations, and have x-rays and scans. Radiotherapy, surgery and chemotherapy are the maintreatments. They are expensive, they are not covered by the National Health Insurance Scheme, they are unsubsidized by the government, and patients have to pay global prices for these services as well as their medication. s. Some insights into how patients who continue treatment manage with the high costs of treatment are provided in the psychosocial analyses of breast cancer treatment by Clegg-Lamptey et al., (2009a). The study of Atobrah, (2006) on aspects of family care for patients with chronic disease further reveal the tremendous support of family members living in industrialized countries for their sick relatives with breast cancer. The ardent desire to keep diagnosis secret was noted in her study as a barrier to access financial help from friends and extended family, compelling such patient to take bank loans at interest rates ranging between 20 percent and 28 percent. Essentially much of the fear and anxieties of patients were related to the heavy financial burden borne by breast cancer patients. More focused qualitative studies on the socio-economic dimensions of breast cancer care and management are needed.

Religious aspects of cancer experiences

Religion plays an important role in the management of complex emotional and psychosocial impact of living with cancer (Opoku et al., 2012; Mayo and Hunter, 2003; Clegg-Lamptey et al., 2009a, 2009b; Atobrah, 2009, 2012). This manifests mainly by patients' attendance at prayer meetings, prayer camps and their participation in relevant activities including fasting, positive confessions, watching and listening to religious programmes and reading of religious literature. The terminal nature of breast cancer makes religion significant, as it may help resolve existential and after-life issues which become imminent in most cases. However, biomedical practitioners have found it problematic when patients' religious beliefs and practices interfere with medical care. The study by Mayo and Hunter (2003) suggests a positive correlation between religious beliefs and notions of fatalism, and ultimately attitudes towards breast cancer screening. Respondents generally believed that events, including breast cancer, are fixed by supernatural beings, and thus they cannot do much about their condition except to commit it to a more powerful supernatural being (God). Their study did not find a significant correlation between education and constructions of fatalism.

Conclusions

It is evident that knowledge gaps exist in social science research on breast cancers in Ghana. Many important themes have not been covered and many questions have not been answered.

Knowledge and awareness remain low and need intensification. There also exists a low level of breast cancer screening practices among Ghanaian women (Opoku et al., 2012). Studies on effective mass communication and adult education approaches and models suitable for increased breast cancer awareness creation and knowledge sharing are needed. Public health promotion approaches could also examine appropriate, culture and context specific communication models to enhance knowledge transition and general communication between patients and health workers, particularly at the time of disease diagnosis, communication of treatment procedures, disease management and prognosis.

Cancer poses a heavy psychological burden and research on all the subfields of psychology is imperative. It is important for instance to understand how patients experience, process and express their feelings at the point of diagnosis and beyond. Areas that require greater research investment include the extent and impact of negative emotions (e.g. fear, guilt, anxiety) that may lead to self-harming practices (including suicide), the nature of grieving among individuals, and the complex process of rationalizing and coping with the experience of cancer. Studies on the psychological impact of cancer on the patients' immediate family, particularly children, are also needed. It may also be important to establish the effects of biomedical therapies, particularly hormonal, on patients' psychological health.

Other critical themes of social science research include understanding and addressing the socio-economic burden of cancer on sufferers and their families, improving health provider-health user relations, and the development of spiritual interventions and palliative care.

References

Agyei Frempong, M.T., Darko, E. and Wiafe Addai, B. (2008). The use of carbohydrate antigen (CA) 15-3 as a tumor marker in detecting breast cancer. *Pakistan Journal of Biological Sciences*; 11(15): 1945-1948.

Aidoo, M. (1973). Some of the types of breast disease at Korle Bu hospital during the period 1968-71 with emphasis on breast cancer- a preliminary study: *Ghana Medical Journal*; 12: 233-236.

de-Graft Aikins, A., Boynton, P. and Atanga, L.L. (2010). Developing effective chronic disease interventions in Africa: insights from Ghana and Cameroon: *Globalisation and Health;* 6(6): 1-15.

Akosa AB, Ampadu FO and Tetteh Y (1999). Male breast cancer in Ghana: *Ghana Medical Journal*; 33(10): 3-8.

Akosa, A.B., Ampadu, F.O. and Tetteh, Y. (2005). Hormone receptor expression in male breast cancers: *Ghana Medical Journal*; 39(1): 14-18.

Anim, J.T. (1979). Breast Diseases- review of surgical material in Korle Bu Hospital (1977- 1978) *Ghana Medical Journal*; 18(1): 30-33.

Antwi, P. and Atobrah, D. (2009). Stigma in the care of people living with HIV/AIDS and cancer in Accra in Oppong C et al (eds.) *Care of the seriously sick and dying: Perspectives from Ghana* (114-149). Norway: BRIC, Unifob Global.

Asumanu, E., Vowotor, R. and Naaeder, S.B. (2000). Pattern of breast disease in Ghana: *Ghana Medical Journal*; 34(4): 206-209.

Atobrah, D. (2009). *Caring for the Chronically Sick within Ga Families: A Case of Traditional Practices and Modern Innovations*. Unpublished Doctoral Dissertation presented to the Institute of African Studies, University of Ghana.

Atobrah, D. (2012). When darkness falls at mid-day: young patients' perceptions and meanings of chronic illness and their implications for medical care: *Ghana Medical Journal;* 46(2): 46-53.

Baako, B.N. and Badoe E.A. (2001). Treatment of breast cancer in Accra: 5-year survival: *Ghana Medical Journal*; 35(2): 90-93.

Bewtra, C. (2010). Clinicopathologic features of female breast cancer in Kumasi, Ghana: *International Journal of Cancer Research*; 6(3): 154-160.

Boyle, P. (2012). Triple – negative breast cancer: epidemiological consideration and recommendations: *Annals of oncology;* 23(6):pvi7-vi12.

Clegg- Lamptey JNA, Aduful K. H, Yarney J, et al (2009). Profile of breast disease at a self- referral clinic in Ghana: *West African Medical Journal*; 28(2):114- 117.

Clegg-Lamptey J, Dakubo J, Attobra YN (2009). Why do breast cancer patients report late or abscond during treatment in Ghana? A pilot study: *Ghana Medical Journal*; 43(3): 127-131.

Clegg-Lamptey, J.NA, Dakubo, J.C.B. Attobra, N. (2009). Psychosocial aspects of breast cancer treatment in Accra, Ghana: *East African Medical Journal*; 86(7): 348-353.

Clegg-Lamptey ,J.N.A., Edusa, C., Ohene Oti, N. et al (2007). Breast cancer risk in patients with breast pain in Accra, Ghana: *East African Medical Journal*; 84(5):215-218.

Clegg-Lamptey, J.N.A., Hodasi, W.M. (2007). A study of breast cancer in Korle-Bu Teaching Hospital: assessing the impact of health education: *Ghana Medical Journal*; 41(2): 72-77.

Ferlay, J.S.H.B.F., Shin, H.R., Bray. F., Forman. D., Mathers, C., Parkin, D.M. (2010). GLOBOCAN 2008, cancer incidence and mortality worldwide: IARC Cancer Base No. 10. *Lyon, France: International Agency for Research on Cancer*, 29.

Field, M.J. (1961). *Religion and Medicine of the Ga People*. Oxford: Oxford University Press.

GLOBOCAN (2004): Cancer incidence, mortality and prevalence: Worldwide Cancer Base. No.5 Lyon, IARC Press.

Helman, Cecil G. (1981). Disease versus illness in general practice. *The Journal of the Royal College of General Practitioners*; 31(230): 548.

Hunter, A., Mayo, R.M. (2003). Fatalism towards breast cancer among the women of Ghana: *Health Care for Women International*; 24(7):606-616.

Kubler-Ross, E., (1969).*On Death and Dying*. NewYork: Macmillan.

Morrow, G. R., & Bellg, A. J. (1994). Behavioral science in translational research and cancer control. *Cancer*, 74(S4), 1409-1417.

Ohene-Yeboah M, Adjei E. (2012). Breast cancer in Kumasi, Ghana: *Ghana Medical Journal*; 46(1): 8-13.

Ohene-Yeboah, M.O.K. (2005). An audit of excised breast lumps in Ghanaian women: *West African Medical Journal*; 24(3): 252-255.

Opoku, S.A, Benwell, M, Yarney, J. (2012). Knowledge, attitudes, beliefs, behavior and breast cancer screening practices in Ghana, West Africa: *Pan African Journal*; 11(28): 1-10.

O'Toole, M. (Ed.). (2003). *Miller-Keane encyclopedia & dictionary of medicine, nursing & allied health*. Philadelphia, Pennsylvania: Elsevier Science, Saunders.

Parkin, D.M, Ferlay J, et al (2004). Cancer in Africa: IARC Lyon: Oxford University Press.

Peiris. L, Alam, N., Agrawal, A. (2012). Tuberculosis of the breast masquerading as breast cancer: *Journal of Surgical Case Reports*; 10(1): 1-3.

Twumasi PA (1975). Medical systems in Ghana: A study of medical sociology: Accra-Tema: Ghana Publishing Corporation.

Quartey-Papafio, J.B (1977). The diagnosis and treatment of early breast cancer: *Ghana Medical Journal*, 16(1) 222-225.

Quartey-Papafio, J.B., Anim, J.T. (1980). Cancer of the breast in Accra: *Ghana Medical Journal*; 19(3), 158-162.

Quartey-Papafio, J.B. (1977). Breast cancer in Accra: *Ghana Medical Journal*;16(3): 189-191.

Quartey-Papafio, J.B. (1978). Primary lymphosarcoma of the breast; a case report 9: *Ghana Medical Journal*;17(3) 183-184.

Stark A, Kleer Celina G, Martin I, et al (2010). African ancestry and higher prevalence of triple breast cancer: *Cancer*; 116(21): 4926-4932.

Tsey, K. (1997). Traditional medicine in contemporary Ghana: A public policy analysis. *Social Science & Medicine*, 45(7), 1065-1074.

Zelle, S.G., Nyarko, K.M., Aikins, A. et al (2012). Costs, effects and cost-effectiveness of breast cancer control in Ghana: *Tropical Medicine & International Health*; 17(8): 1031-1043.

Chapter 5

A review of epidemiological studies of asthma in Ghana[1]

Abena S. Amoah, Audrey G. Forson and Daniel A. Boakye

Introduction

Defining the disease

Asthma is a chronic disease characterised by recurrent attacks of breathlessness and wheezing which vary in severity as well as frequency (WHO, 2008). Allergic asthma is the most common form of the disease with symptoms being triggered by environmental antigens known as allergens (AAAI, 2008). These allergens activate sub-mucosal mast cells in the lower airways of the respiratory tract leading to de-granulation, secretion of inflammatory mediators, bronchial smooth muscle contraction and eventually to reversible airway obstruction (Parham, 2005). Non-allergic asthma (also referred to as 'intrinsic asthma') usually occurs later in life and is not associated with allergic triggers (Corrigan, 2004). Individuals suffering from this particular condition are often females and are more likely to have sinus polyps (Romanet-Manent et al., 2002).

Global Burden of Asthma

The World Health Organization (WHO) estimates that there are 300 million people world-wide suffering from asthma. In fact, over the past few decades, there has been a dramatic rise in the global incidence of the disease ,particularly in industrialised nations (Braman, 2006). This phenomenon, which has sometimes been described as the 'asthma epidemic' (Maziak, 2005), has come with a huge economic burden world-wide as a result of significant healthcare utilisation associated with this chronic condition (Bahadori et al., 2009).

Recent studies indicate that asthma is not just a public health problem for developed countries but is increasingly becoming widespread in the developing

---

1 Previously published as Amoah, A.S., Forson, A.G., and D.A. Boakye, D.A. (2012).Risk factors for asthma in Ghana: a review. *Ghana Medical Journal*, 46(2), 23-28.

world. Sub-Saharan African countries are no exceptions. A recent survey of asthma and allergies in childhood found that the prevalence of asthma symptoms among children in Kenya was 15.1 percent, in Nigeria 13.0 percent and in South Africa 20.3 percent (Wijst and Boakye, 2007).

Aetiology of asthma

Asthma is often described as a complex condition with no single biological marker and multiple aetiological causes (Sears, 1997). Its development is seen as an intricate interaction between genetic and environmental factors (Martinez, 1997). Indeed, a number of novel candidate genes and pathways in the pathogenesis of asthma have been identified (Hansel and Diette, 2007). Exposures to environmental triggers that may predispose towards early childhood asthma start from *in utero*. An example of one such risk factor is maternal smoking during pregnancy (Kumar, 2008). Furthermore, studies indicate that atopy, the genetic tendency to develop Immunoglobulin E (IgE) antibodies in response to an allergen (Arshad et al., 2001), is an important factor in asthma aetiology (Arbes et al., 2007). During infancy, for example, exposures to housedust mite, animal dander or pollen in predisposed individuals can increase their risk of developing asthma. However, in recent years, new evidence suggests that wheezing episodes associated with asthma may also be caused by respiratory viral infections (Le Souef, 2009). This is a direct challenge to the widely-accepted paradigm that childhood asthma is an atopic disease (Le Souef, 2009).

Other risk factors for asthma include: family history of the disease (Litonjua et al., 1998), consumption of a diet with reduced antioxidants (Devereux and Seaton, 2003; Allen et al., 2009), obesity (Sin et al., 2008), residence in inner-city urban areas (Bryant-Stephens, 2009) and also reduced exposure to childhood infections as postulated in the 'hygiene hypothesis' (Strachan, 1989). According to this hypothesis, declining family sizes, higher standards of cleanliness and reduced exposure to childhood infections were responsible for the dramatic increase in allergic disorders in industrialised countries (Strachan, 1989). Since then, a number of investigations have sought to explore the link between parasitic infections and the development of asthma and other allergies (Yazdanbakhsh et al., 2002). Helminth infections are of particular interest since both helminths and allergic diseases are associated with strong T-helper type 2 (TH2) cell-mediated immune responses (Yazdanbakhsh et al., 2001).

One theory is that susceptibility to allergic diseases in developed countries represents the manifestation of a phenotype that evolved specifically to deal with a helminth-endemic environment which requires strong TH-2 driven responses and in the absence of helminths, the immune system never develops immune tolerance leading to a predisposition towards allergic disease (Flohr et al., 2009).

Burden of asthma in Ghana

At present, there is insufficient data on the current burden of asthma in Ghana. However, anecdotal clinical reports and surveys among schoolchildren indicate that asthma is an important cause of childhood morbidity in the country especially in urban areas (Forson et al., 2006). Aside from a deficiency in information on the overall prevalence of asthma in Ghana and whether it is largely of allergic or non-allergic origin, there are also a number of challenges that have hampered an effective response to the disease.[26] Such challenges include difficulties in the diagnosis of the condition and a lack of knowledge on asthma management guidelines (Hesse, 1995). There has also been inadequate uniformity in asthma treatment in Ghanaian healthcare institutions given that the focus tends to be on acute symptom management (crisis management) instead of chronic disease care (Forson et al., 2006).

Despite challenges, there have been some developments in the field of asthma research in Ghana that have enriched our understanding of the disease. In this review, we examine the available literature on asthma epidemiological studies conducted in Ghana and what these reveal about the disease in the country. We also explore how these investigations fit into the wider context of findings from other parts of sub-Saharan Africa and the world.

Epidemiological studies of asthma in Ghana

Atopy and Asthma

Studies exploring the association between atopic sensitisation and asthma in Ghana date back to the first published study on asthma in the country. In 1973, Commey and Haddock published their findings on a hospital-based investigation in which adult asthmatics in the capital city, Accra, were skin prick tested for atopic sensitisation. They found that 33 percent of 40 individuals with doctor-diagnosed asthma were sensitised to house dust mite extracts (Commey and Haddock, 1973).

Twenty years later in 1993, Addo-Yobo and colleagues also explored the association between asthma and atopic sensitisation. However, they focused on children in the city of Kumasi in the Ashanti Region as well as children in a rural community in the same region. They conducted an investigation in which exercise testing was used to explore the prevalence of exercise-induced bronchospasm (EIB). An exercise challenge is just one method used to confirm an asthma diagnosis and provides an objective indicator that has been utilised in epidemiological studies across the globe (O'Byrne et al., 2009). As part of their study, a total of 1,095 schoolchildren aged between 9-16 years underwent exercise challenges. Additionally, a total of 916 children were skin-prick tested for atopic sensitisation to a panel of allergens that included house dustmite extracts and pet allergens. The authors found the prevalence of EIB was 3.1 percent while atopic sensitisation was 4.4 percent (Addo-Yobo et al., 1997). They also observed no significant differences in the prevalence of atopy between children with EIB and those without. Addo-Yobo et al., (1997) concluded that this could also be as a result of inadequate power due to the small number of children with EIB.

This investigation demonstrates the significance of EIB as an objective indicator of asthma. However, in a subsequent study conducted in the wet season five months after their initial investigation (among the same group of children), Addo-Yobo et al., observed an effect of seasonal variability associated with EIB (Addo-Yobo et al., 2002). They found that the prevalence of EIB reduced from 3.1 percent (dry season) to 1.55 percent (wet season) and concluded that the value of EIB may be limited by environmental factors such as temperature, humidity and air pollution(Addo-Yobo et al., 2002). They also reasoned that the results obtained during the dry season were a more accurate reflection of 'true' EIB prevalence than during the wet season.

In a 10-year follow-up to their 1993 study, Addo-Yobo et al., re-examined the prevalence of EIB as an asthma marker following the same methodology in the same study schools. Their subsequent investigation established that the prevalence of EIB had increased from 3.1 percent to 5.2 percent while atopic sensitisation had also doubled over the 10 year period (Addo-Yobo et al., 2007). A notable finding of this later study was that atopic sensitisation was now significantly associated with EIB. Specifically, atopy was linked with a two-fold increase in the risk of EIB (OR=2.10, 95 percent CI 1.29 – 3.42, p=0.003) (Addo-Yobo et al., 2007). This suggests that as time went on, there was a transition from largely non-allergic EIB to more allergic EIB within this population. This transition could have been driven by lifestyle changes associated with development.

Other EIB studies from various parts of Africa have made similar observations (Perzanowski et al., 2002; Calvert, 2005). An investigation from Kenya found a strong relationship between EIB and atopy, determined by both IgE antibodies (p=0.02) and skin-prick testing (p=0.002), in urban children (mean age, 11 years). In contrast, out of 13 rural participants in this study who had EIB, none were skin prick test positive (Perzanowski et al., 2002). These findings further support the notion that the relationship between atopy and asthma is driven by factors associated with urbanisation in sub-Saharan Africa.

A recent study on international variations in asthma symptom prevalence amongst children has also provided insights into the association between atopy and asthma in Ghana. This investigation was part of the International Study of Asthma and Allergy in Childhood (ISAAC) Phase II and involved the participation of 30 study sites in 22 countries. One selected centre was the rural town of Kintampo in the Brong-Ahafo Region of Ghana. The ISAAC Phase II methodology involved the use of a standardised parental questionnaire on symptoms of asthma among children aged between 8 and 12 years as well as skin prick testing for atopic sensitization (Weinmayr et al, 2007). The Ghana study collected questionnaire data for a total of 1,354 children of whom 1,322 were skin prick tested (Weinmayr et al., 2007). Out of the 30 centres across the globe, the prevalence of skin reactivity to at least one allergen (atopy) was lowest in Kintampo (1.7 percent) and highest in Hong Kong (45.3 percent)(Weinmayr et al., 2007). The ISAAC team also found that the overall prevalence of reported wheeze in Kintampo was 6.4 percent while the percentage of those with 'atopic wheeze' (defined by reported wheeze within the past year coupled with a positive skin prick test) was 0.3 percent. Furthermore, 'non-atopic wheeze' (defined by reported wheeze without a positive skin prick test) in Kintampo was determined to be 6.2 percent thus illustrating that most of the observed wheeze had non-atopic origins. This observation supports the hypothesis that some wheezing episodes often associated with asthma may be caused by factors other than allergy such as respiratory viral infections (Le Souef, 2009). Unfortunately, the ISAAC study did not explore this possibility. Moreover, the study did not include an urban site in Ghana to compare the prevalence of reported wheeze and also to determine whether this could be attributed more to atopy than in the rural study centre.

The ISAAC Phase II investigation also explored the relationships between gross national income (GNI) per capita (for each study country), atopy and asthma symptoms. It was determined that the association between skin-prick test reactivity and wheeze was statistically significant in almost all the affluent countries examined. In countries with high GNIs, skin-prick test reactivity was associated with a 4-fold increase in the risk of wheeze (OR=4.0, 95 percent CI 3.5 – 4.6) while this was much weaker in non-affluent countries (OR=2.0, 95 percent CI 1.5 – 3.3) (Weinmayr et al., 2007). In a recent review of allergic disorders in Africa, Obeng and colleagues hypothesize that in countries with high GNIs, there is a strong relationship between allergen-specific IgE, skin reactivity to allergens and the manifestations of allergic disorders like asthma. On the other hand, in countries with low GNIs (such as Ghana), these relationships become less strong and are even weaker in rural than in urban areas (Obeng et al., 2008). According to the hypothesis, one would expect that in urban areas in a country such as Ghana, there is likely to be more asthma of allergic origins compared to rural areas. However the exact mechanisms behind these differences remain unknown.

Urban-rural gradient, socioeconomic status differences and asthma

A significant observation of asthma epidemiological studies conducted in Ghana has been the marked differences in the asthma phenotype between urban and rural populations. Additionally, key variations within urban areas based on socioeconomic groupings have also been noted. From their EIB study conducted in 1993, Addo-Yobo et al., found that among children attending what they classified as an 'urban rich' school, the prevalence of EIB was highest (4.2 percent) compared to 'urban poor' and rural schools (Addo-Yobo et al., 1997). Ten years later, the EIB prevalence among these urban affluent children had doubled to 8.3 percent (Addo-Yobo et al., 2007) while among urban poor children it changed from 1.4 percent (1993) to 3.0 percent in (2003) and among rural children from 2.2 percent (1993) to 3.9 percent (2003). It is also noteworthy that the prevalence of EIB among urban poor people was not much different from (and even lower than) prevalence among rural children. The authors rationalise this by explaining that differences in EIB may reflect varying lifestyles rather than areas of residence. The prevalence of skin-prick sensitisation to any allergen was also highest in urban rich children followed by urban poor and finally rural children. This reinforces the concept of a more affluent lifestyle being associated with allergic sensitisation.

These studies demonstrate the importance of an urban-rural gradient as well as socioeconomic differences in the prevalence of markers for asthma in Ghana. Similar trends have been observed in other parts of Africa (Obeng et al., 2008; Weinberg, 2000). For example, Odhiambo et al., (1998) found a much lower prevalence of questionnaire-derived markers of asthma among rural than among urban children in Kenya. Moreover, another investigation conducted by the same group also observed a higher prevalence of EIB in Kenyan urban children than among rural children (Ng'ang'a et al., 1998). Therefore, urbanisation and related lifestyle factors appear to be contributing significantly to differences in the prevalence of asthma and allergies across Africa. However, as Obeng et al., (2008) point out in their review, there is a need to clearly define 'rural' and 'urban' in epidemiological studies of allergies across the continent. Identifying the specific factors within urban environments that may be behind the increasing prevalence of asthma and other allergic disorders is indeed an arduous but necessary task.

Environmental risk factors and asthma

There has been a plethora of studies that have explored environmental risk factors for asthma but less from sub-Saharan Africa and fewer still from Ghana. Addo-Yobo et al., (2001) conducted a case-control study among urban schoolchildren in Kumasi to examine such risk factors. As part of this investigation, 50 asthmatic children aged 9 to16 years were matched by age and sex to randomly selected healthy controls attending the same schools as cases. The risk factors for asthma examined included sensitisation to environmental allergens, Immunoglobulin E (IgE) measurements, sibship position, inner-city residence, allergen levels in households, dog ownership as well as the use of electricity for cooking. From multivariate analysis, the authors found that being asthmatic was significantly associated with sensitisation to house dust mite and cockroach allergens, inner-city residence as well as having a sibship position less than five (Addo-Yobo et al., 2001).

This study further demonstrates the importance of atopic sensitisation as a risk factor for asthma in urban Ghana. Sibship position was used as a proxy measure for exposure to more infections since, according to the 'hygiene hypothesis', fewer siblings means fewer infections and perhaps more allergies (Strachan, 2000).

Residence in an inner-city environment has long been associated with asthma, particularly in relation to living in inner-city areas of the United States (Bryant-Stephens, 2009) where there is likely to be greater exposures to irritants (e.g. tobacco smoke), pollutants (such as diesel-related particles) and indoor allergens (Wright et al., 2007). Addo-Yobo et al., postulated that although unclear, inner-city residence as a risk factor for asthma in an African city may be related to pollution from automobile fumes, over-crowding, dampness, modern buildings and furnishings that promote indoor allergens (Addo-Yobo et al., 2001). However, they did note that their proxy measures for over-crowding were not associated with asthma in their study. Moreover, the levels of traffic-related pollutants in Kumasi were not measured so the potential contribution of such pollutants to asthma in this study remains unknown.

Exposure to traffic-related pollutants, especially emissions from motor vehicles, has been linked to the increase in asthma in industrialised countries based on findings from animal model experiments and human exposure studies (Morgensten et al., 2008). These have shown that pollutants such as diesel exhaust particles can induce the development of allergic immune responses and enhance allergic inflammation (Heinrich and Wichman, 2004). However, there have been conflicting findings from studies conducted in Europe, with some showing a positive correlation between traffic-related pollutants and asthma while others observe no effect (Heinrich and Wichman, 2004). Although the reasons behind inconsistencies in observations remain unclear, they may be related to differences in indicators used in the varying studies and how these were measured.

Only a couple of studies of traffic-related asthma have been conducted in Africa. One investigation from an urban area in Ethiopia conducted among 7,609 children and adults observed that living in close proximity to road vehicle traffic was related to an increase in the risk of wheeze but other environmental factors were also likely to play a role (Venn et al., 2005). Unfortunately, no investigations into traffic-related pollutants have been done in Ghana to establish the extent to which these may be contributing to the observed increase in the incidence of asthma in the country. Therefore, this remains an essential direction for future studies on asthma in Ghana.

With regard to indoor allergen levels, Addo-Yobo and colleagues (2001) found that house dust mite allergens were in abundance in both the homes of cases and controls but were significantly higher among asthmatics compared to controls (p<0.05). This observation, along with the fact that there was greater atopic sensitisation to dust mites among asthmatics, further demonstrates the importance of house dust mites in asthma aetiology in Ghana. Some research has been done on the distribution and abundance of house dust mite species in homes in the Greater Accra Region of Ghana that complement these observations (Anokye-Danso, 2001; Obeng, 2001; Larbi, 2003). Surveys conducted found high house dust mite densities within houses, especially in stuffed furniture and carpets. They also observed the predominance of *Dermatophagoides* mite species (Anokye-Danso, 2001; Obeng, 2001; Larbi, 2003) which have been implicated in asthma aetiology world-wide (Huss et al., 2001). Although these mite distribution studies did not explore asthma prevalence, they do provide some indications of elevated levels of indoor allergens that may be associated with asthma within Ghanaian homes. Furthermore, the fact that certain household furnishings (associated with affluence) were identified as house dust mite reservoirs provides additional support for the hypothesis that particular lifestyle factors may be associated with the increasing prevalence of asthma in Ghana.

One environmental factor that was not found to be associated with increased risk of asthma from the case-control study by Addo-Yobo et al., was exposure to allergens from pets such as dogs. A recent meta-analysis of studies from across the globe on asthma and exposure to furry pets found that dog ownership increased the risk of the disease while cat ownership exerted a slight protective effect against asthma (Takkouche et al., 2008). Given the link between pet allergen sensitisation and asthma, an investigation examining pet allergen levels in homes in Kumasi, (Ghana) compared to homes in Manchester, (United Kingdom) was conducted and published in 2001. In this study, Woodcock et al., (2001) observed that cat and /or dog ownership rates in Ghana and the UK were similar. However, they also found that levels of pet allergens within Ghanaian homes were 75 times lower for dogs and 275 times lower for cats than in UK homes with pets. The authors concluded that similar proportions in pet ownership in different countries cannot be equated with similar levels of exposure to pet allergens. This would be expected since pets in Ghana are more likely to be kept outdoors given that dogs are maintained for security purposes and cats largely for the control of domestic rodents (Woodcock et al., 2001). However, it would be interesting to investigate if lifestyle changes associated with Westernisation could be impacting on pet ownership dynamics in Ghana and perhaps leading to higher levels of indoor pet allergens.

An emergent environmental issue in Ghana that may potentially impact on the development of asthma and allergies is exposure to toxic material from electronic waste known as e-waste. Over the past couple of years there have been some reports on the shipping of electronic waste (often old computers) from industrialised countries to African countries including Ghana (Ross, 2008). This e-waste is contains toxic metals such as lead, cadmium, mercury and old plastic casing that when burned in public landfill sites releases carcinogenic dioxins and polyaromatic hydrocarbons into the atmosphere (Schmidt, 2006). Polyaromatic hydrocarbons in particular have been linked to the induction of asthma symptoms (Schneider et al., 2005) but very little research has been done on this subject. Indeed, the health effects of e-waste on individuals in African countries such as Ghana have not been explored by formal studies and present a pertinent research direction.

Heredity, early life risk factors and asthma

A number of asthma research studies have reported a strong correlation between family history of asthma and increased risk of the disease (Sears, 1997). Addo-Yobo and colleagues explored this in their study on asthma risk factors in urban Ghana. From univariate analysis, they found that 'asthma in one's family', 'paternal asthma', 'having a second-degree relative with asthma' were all associated with doctor-diagnosed asthma but not maternal asthma (Addo-Yobo et al., 2001). However, after adjusting for confounding, none of these variables remained associated with the disease.

In recent years, the Noguchi Memorial Institute for Medical Research (NMIMR) Asthma and Allergies group has explored atopic sensitisation in rural as well as urban children in the Greater Accra Region of Ghana. One study we conducted on risk factors for asthma among 431 schoolchildren examined family history of the disease and also some early life factors associated with asthma (Amoah et al., 2007). We used a questionnaire adapted from the ISAAC Phase II study modules to determine the prevalence of asthma. After adjusting for confounders and taking clustering within families into account, we observed that reported asthma was strongly associated with maternal asthma (OR=3.69, 95 percent CI 1.71 -7.94, p=0.001) as well as breastfeeding duration for less than six months (OR=5.26, 95 percent CI 1.60 -18.71, p=0.005). Aside from a relatively small sample size, a limitation of our study was the use of a questionnaire as a measurement tool since this may have introduced some degree of information bias into our findings. Nevertheless, other research studies have observed that maternal asthma significantly increases the risk of asthma in offspring although the exact mechanisms through which this occurs remain unknown. Furthermore, murine models implicate the cytokine interleukin 4 (IL-4) and maternal environmental exposures in maternal transmission of asthma risk (Lim and Kobzik, 2009).

The role of breastfeeding duration in asthma aetiology remains a controversial area of research with studies showing varying findings. Some report no effect of prolonged breastfeeding on asthma (Duncan and Sears, 2008) while others point to a protective effect (Oddy et al., 1999; Scholtens et al., 2009). A few investigations have also demonstrated an increased asthma risk associated with longer breastfeeding (Chan-Yeung and Becker, 2006). Dagoye et al (2004) found that longer breastfeeding duration corresponded to an increased risk of reported wheeze among Ethiopian children living in an urban area. On the other hand, studies conducted among Kenyan children found no association between breastfeeding duration (less than six months) and EIB (Ng'ang'a et al., 1998) or breastfeeding duration and symptom markers of asthma (i.e. shortness of breath with 'wheeze ever') (Odhiambo et al., 1998). In light of contrasting findings, more research is needed to explore in-depth the role of breastfeeding duration and other early life factors on the development of asthma in sub-Saharan Africa.

Parasitic infections and asthma

Few publications from Ghana have examined the link between parasitic infections and asthma. In their case-control study on asthma risk factors among urban children, Addo-Yobo et al., (2001) collected stool samples to detect the presence of the helminths *Ascaris lumbricoides* and *Schistosoma mansoni*. However, no conclusions could be reached due to the low numbers of parasite-positive samples.

With regard to other studies from across the globe, a systematic review that examined current parasitic infection and risk of asthma or wheeze found that after adjusting for confounders, hookworm infection had an overall protective effect against asthma (pooled OR=0.50, 95 percent CI 0.28 – 0.90, p=0.02) (Leonardi et al., 2006). Interestingly, the review established that *A. lumbricoides* infection appeared to increase the risk of asthma (OR=1.34, 95 percent CI 1.05 – 1.71, p=0.02). The fact that these risk effects act in opposite directions demonstrates that different intestinal helminths may act through dissimilar mechanisms. Therefore, elucidating the specific immune pathways involved has been an important focus of recent research studies.

A newly published investigation from Brazil identified specific co-stimulatory molecules that may be involved in the down-regulation of inflammatory allergic responses among asthmatics infected with the helminth *Schistosoma mansoni* compared to un-infected controls (Oliveira et al,. 2009). This study has particular relevance to Ghana since schistosomiasis remains endemic in some parts of the country (Nsowah-Nuamah et al., 2001). One recent publication from the NMIMR Asthma and Allergies group observed that among schoolchildren residing in a rural area of the Greater Accra Region, the helminth *Schistosoma haematobium* suppressed the expression of certain genes associated with asthma (Hartgers et al., 2008). The specific genes examined were Toll-like receptor-2 (TLR-2) and suppressor of cytokine signalling-3 (SOCS-3). In this investigation, the inhibition of these genes was also associated with lower atopic sensitisation. Specific TLR-2 gene polymorphisms have been also been linked to reduced asthma prevalence in other studies (Yang et al., 2006). In addition, murine models show that the SOCS-3 expression is associated with TH2 cell responses and multiple pathological features of asthma in an airway hypersensitivity model system (Seki et al., 2003) Therefore, our research provides further evidence that helminth infections may suppress specific genes that are involved in asthma aetiology leading to a lower prevalence of the disease among populations in helminth-endemic areas. The exact mechanism through which this may occur remains unclear and consequently more investigations are needed.

Conclusions and future directions

Epidemiological studies of asthma in Ghana demonstrate that there is an increasing prevalence of the disease, specifically among children. Investigations also show evidence of an association between atopic sensitisation and asthma symptoms with this effect being strongest in urban areas. Research conducted illustrates the value of exercise challenges and exercise-induced bronchospasm (EIB) in generating an objective indicator of asthma. However, there are also indications that EIB is affected by seasonal variation. Consistent with findings from other parts of sub-Saharan Africa and the world, environmental allergens such as house dust mite and cockroach are significant in asthma aetiology in

Ghana. Findings from Ghana also show that exposure to pet allergen levels may not be important in the development of asthma in this country in contrast to studies from the developed world.

Investigations have also demonstrated the implications of urban-rural differences as well as socioeconomic status in asthma aetiology. Inner-city residence may be of significance but it is still unclear which factors in Ghanaian inner-city areas may be associated with asthma. Future studies are needed to explore the urban-rural gradient in-depth as well as socio-economic factors associated with asthma. There is very little information available on the effects of environmental air pollutants derived from motor vehicle traffic as well as combusted electronic waste on asthma in Ghana or even other parts of Africa. Both these areas represent pertinent directions for prospective asthma research.

Early life risk factors and heredity have been found to be important in asthma aetiology in Ghana but again, more work is needed in this area. Recent studies in Ghana implicate helminth infections in the suppression of allergic sensitisation and perhaps even inhibition of asthma but this is yet to be investigated in-depth. Advances in technology such as the use of molecular immunological techniques may be vital in future investigations of asthma in Ghana to elucidate the immunological mechanisms by which helminth infections may protect against the disease.

An area of research severely lacking in Ghana are that of studies on asthma patient care, patient experiences and even perceptions of asthma. In addition, there are no investigations that quantify the economic burden of asthma on individual patients on the Ghanaian economy. These analyses are essential as the country strives towards universal health coverage under the National Health Insurance Scheme (NHIS). Moreover, skin-prick testing for allergic sensitisation would greatly complement asthma diagnostic services in Ghana. This would allow the differentiation between allergic and non-allergic asthma to be made and thus aid in the provision of appropriate individual treatment of the disease. Such initiatives alongside surveys on risk factors for asthma are imperative if we are to avert an asthma epidemic in a rapidly urbanising developing country such as Ghana.

References

Addo-Yobo, E.O.D., Custovic, A., Taggart. S.C.O., Asafo-Agyei, A.P., Woodcock. A. (1997).Exercise induced bronchospasm in Ghana: differences in prevalence between urban and rural schoolchildren. *Thorax* **52**(2):161-5.

Addo-Yobo, E.O.D., Custovic. A., Taggart, S.C.O., Craven, M., Bonnie, B. and Woodcock, A. (2001). Risk factors for asthma in urban Ghana. *Journal of Allergy and Clinical Immunology*. **108**(3):363-368.

Addo-Yobo, E.O.D., Custovic, A., Taggart, S.C.O., Asafo-Agyei. A.P. and Woodcock. A. (2002).Seasonal variability in exercise test responses in Ghana. *Pediatr Allergy Immunol*. **13**:303-306.

Addo-Yobo, E.O.D., Woodcock, A., Allotey, A., Baffoe-Bonnie, B., Strachan. D. and Custovic, A. (2007). Exercise-Induced Bronchospasm and Atopy in Ghana: Two Surveys Ten Years Apart. *PLoS Medicine*. **4**(2):e70.

Allen, S., Britton, J.R., Leonardi-Bee, J.A. (2009). Association between antioxidant vitamins and asthma outcome measures: systematic review and meta-analysis. *Thorax*. **64**(7):610-619.

AAAI. Topic of the Month - March - Is your asthma allergic?: American Academy of Allergy, Asthma and Immunology (AAAI), 2008.

Amoah, A.S., Obeng, B.B., Larbi, I.A. et al. Risk Factors for Asthma among School Children in the Greater Accra Region of Ghana. Paper presented *at the 1st Annual Workshop, British Academy UK-Africa Academic Partnership on Chronic Disease in Africa, Noguchi Memorial Institute for Medical Research*, Accra Ghana.

Anokye-Danso, F. (2001). Variations in the Populations of House Dust Mite Species, B.Sc. Thesis: Department of Zoology, University of Ghana. 86 pages.

Arbes, S.J., Gergen, P.J., Vaughn. B., Zeldin, D.C. (2007). Asthma cases attributable to atopy: Results from the Third National Health and Nutrition Examination Survey. *The Journal of allergy and clinical immunology*. **120**(5):1139-1145.

Arshad, S.H., Tariq, S.M., Matthews. S., Hakim. E. (2001) Sensitization to Common Allergens and Its Association With Allergic Disorders at Age 4 Years: A Whole Population Birth Cohort Study. *Pediatrics*. **108**(2):E33.

Bahadori, K., Doyle-Waters. M., Marra. C. et al. (2009). Economic burden of asthma: a systematic review. *BMC Pulmonary Medicine*. **9**(1):24.

Braman, S.S. (2006). The Global Burden of Asthma. *Chest*. **130**(1_suppl):4S-12.

Bryant-Stephens, T. (2009). Asthma disparities in urban environments. *The Journal of allergy and clinical immunology*. **123**(6):1199-1206.

Calvert, Burney. (2005). Effect of body mass on exercise-induced bronchospasm and atopy in African children. *Journal of Allergy and Clinical Immunology*. **116**(4):773-779.

Chan-Yeung, M., and Becker A. (2006).Primary prevention of childhood asthma and allergic disorders. *Curr Opin Allergy Clin Immunol.* **6**(3):146-51

Commey, J, Haddock, D.R.W. (1973).Skin Sensitivity to House Dust Mite Extracts in Ghanaian Asthmatics in Accra. *Trans Roy Soc Trop Med Hyg.* **67**(1):109-11.

Corrigan, C. (2004). Mechanisms of intrinsic asthma. *Curr Opin Allergy Clin Immunol.* **4**(1):53-6.

Dagoye, D. Bekele, Z., Woldemichael, K. et al. (2004). Domestic risk factors for wheeze in urban and rural Ethiopian children. *QJM.* **97**(8):489-498.

Devereux, G. and Seaton, A. (2005). Diet as a risk factor for atopy and asthma. *The Journal of allergy and clinical immunology.* **115**(6):1109-1117.

Duncan, J.M. and Sears, M. R. (2008). Breastfeeding and allergies: time for a change in paradigm? *Curr Opin Allergy Clin Immunol.* **8**(5):398-405.

Flohr, C., Quinnell. R.J.and Britton, J. (2009). Do helminth parasites protect against atopy and allergic disease? *C.linical & Experimental Allergy.* **39**(1):20-32.

Forson, A., Addo-Yobo. E.O., Arhin. P. (2006). Strategic Plan for Asthma, NCD Ministry of Health, Ghana.

Hanse,l. N.N. and Diette, G.B.. (2007) Gene Expression Profiling in Human Asthma. *Proc Am Thorac Soc.* **4**(1):32-36.

Hartgers, F.C., Obeng, B.B., Kruize, Y.C.M. et al.(2008). Lower Expression of TLR2 and SOCS-3 Is Associated with Schistosoma haematobium Infection and with Lower Risk for Allergic Reactivity in Children Living in a Rural Area in Ghana. *PLoS Negl Trop Dis* **2**(4):e227.

Heinrich, J. and Wichmann, H-E. (2004). Traffic related pollutants in Europe and their effect on allergic disease. *Current Opinion in Allergy and Clinical Immunology* . **4**(5):341-348.

Hesse, I. (1995). Knowledge of asthma and its management in newly qualified doctors in Accra, Ghana. *Respir Med.* **89**(1):35-9.

Huss, K., Adkinson, N.F., Eggleston, P.A., Dawson, C., Van Natta, M.L., Hamilton. R.G. (2001). House dust mite and cockroach exposure are strong risk factors for positive allergy skin test responses in the Childhood Asthma Management Program*. *The Journal of allergy and clinical immunology.* **107**(1):48-54.

Kumar, R.(2008). Prenatal factors and the development of asthma. *Curr Opin Pediatr.* **20**(6):682-7.

Larbi, I.A. (2003). Studies on the Distribution and Abundance of House Dust Mite Species, B.Sc. Thesis: Department of Zoology, University of Ghana. 71 pages.

Leonardi-Bee, J., Pritchard, D., Britton, J. (2006). the Parasites in Asthma C. Asthma and Current Intestinal Parasite Infection: Systematic Review and Meta-Analysis. *Am. J. Respir. Crit. Care Med.* **174**(5):514-523.

Le Souëf, P. (2009). Gene-environmental interaction in the development of atopic asthma: new developments. *Curr opin Allergy Clin Immunol.* **9**(2):123-7.

Lim, R.H.and Kobzik, L.(2009). Maternal Transmission of Asthma Risk. *American Journal of Reproductive Immunology.* **61**(1):1-10.

Litonjua Augusto, A., Carey. Vincent, J., Burge Harriet, A., Weiss Scott, T, Gold Diane, R. (1998). Parental History and the Risk for Childhood Asthma . Does Mother Confer More Risk than Father? *Am. J. Respir. Crit. Care Med.* **158**(1):176-181.

Martinez, F. (1997). Complexities of the Genetics of Asthma. *Am. J. Respir. Crit. Care Med.* **156**(4):117S-122.

Maziak, W. (2005). The Asthma Epidemic and our Artificial Habitats. *BMC Pulmonary Medicine.* **5**(1):5.

Morgenstern, V., Zutavern, A., Cyrys. J. et al. (2008).Atopic Diseases, Allergic Sensitization, and Exposure to Traffic-related Air Pollution in Children. *Am. J. Respir. Crit. Care Med.* **177**(12):1331-1337.

Ng'ang'a, L.W., Odhiambo, J.A., Mungai, M.W. et al. (1998). Prevalence of exercise induced bronchospasm in Kenyan school children: an urban-rural comparison. *Thorax.* **53**(11):919-926.

Nsowah-Nuamah, N., Mensah, G., Aryeetey. M., Wagatsuma, Y., Bentil, G. (2001). Urinary schistosomiasis in southern Ghana: a logistic regression approach to data from a community-based integrated control program. *Am J Trop Med Hyg* **65**(5):484-490.

Obeng, B.B.(2001). Preliminary Studies of the Distribution of Dust Mite Species; B.Sc. Thesis: Department of Zoology; University of Ghana. 86 pages.

Obeng, B.B., Hartgers, F., Boakye,D., Yazdanbakhsh. M.(2008). Out of Africa: what can be learned from the studies of allergic disorders in Africa and Africans? *Current Opinion in Allergy and Clinical Immunology.* **8**(5):391-397 10.1097/ACI.0b013e32830ebb70.

O' Byrne, P.M., Gauvreau, G.M.,and Brannan, J.D. (2009). Provoked models of asthma: what have we learnt? *Clinical & Experimental Allergy.* **39**(2):181-192.

Oddy, W.H., Holt. P.G., Sly. P.D. et al. (1999). Association between breast feeding and asthma in 6 year old children: findings of a prospective birth cohort study. *BMJ.* **319**(7213):815-819.

Odhiambo, J., Ng'ang'a. L., Mungai, M. et al. (1998). Urban-rural differences in questionnaire-derived markers of asthma in Kenyan school children. *Eur Respir J.* **12**(5):1105-1112.

Oliveira, R.R., Gollob, K.J., Figueiredo, J.P. et al. (2009). Schistosoma mansoni infection alters co-stimulatory molecule expression and cell activation in asthma. *Microbes and Infection.* **11**(2):223-229.

Parham, P. (2005).The Immune System. 2nd ed. New York Garland Science.

Perzanowsk, M.S., Ng'ang'a, L.W., Carter, M.C. et al. (2002). Atopy, asthma, and antibodies to Ascaris among rural and urban children in Kenya. *The Journal of pediatrics.* **140**(5):582-588.

Romanet-Manent, S., Charpin. D., Magnan. A., Lanteaume. A., Vervloet. D. (2002). Allergic vs nonallergic asthma: what makes the difference? *Allergy.* **57**(7):607-613.

Ross, W. (2008).Ghana's growing e-waste trade. BBC News Online.

Sears, M.R. (1997). Epidemiology of Childhood Asthma. *Lancet* . **350**:1015-1020.

Scholtens, S., Wijga, A.H., Brunekreef, B., et al. (2009). Breast feeding, parental allergy and asthma in children followed for 8 years. The PIAMA birth cohort study. *Thorax.* **64**(7):604-609.

Schmidt, C.W. (2006)> Unfair Trade e-Waste in Africa. *Environ Health Perspect* **114**(4):232-235.

Schneider, J.C., Card. G.L., Pfau. J.C., Holian. A. (2005). Air Pollution Particulate SRM 1648 Causes Oxidative Stress in RAW 264.7 Macrophages Leading to Production of Prostaglandin E2, a Potential Th2 Mediator. *Inhalation Toxicology.* **17**(14):871-877.

Seki, Y., Inoue. H., Nagata. N. et al. (2003). SOCS-3 regulates onset and maintenance of TH2-mediated allergic responses. *Nat Med.* **9**(8):1047-1054.

Sin, D.D., Sutherland. E.R. 92008). Obesity and the lung: 4. Obesity and asthma. *Thorax.* **63**(11):1018-1023.

Strachan DP. (1989). Hayfever, hygiene and household size. *BMJ* . (299):1259-60.

Strachan, D. (2000). Family size, infection and atopy: the first decade of the "hygiene hypothesis". *Thorax.* **55**(Suppl 1):S1-S10.

Takkouche, B., González-Barcala. F.J., Etminan. M., FitzGerald, M. (2008). Exposure to furry pets and the risk of asthma and allergic rhinitis: a meta-analysis. *Allergy***63**(7):857-864.

Venn, A., Yemaneberhan, H., Lewis, S., Parry, E., Britton. J. (2005). Proximity of the home to roads and the risk of wheeze in an Ethiopian population. *Occup Environ Med.* **62**(6):376-380.

Weinberg, E.G. (2000). Urbanization and childhood asthma: an African perspective. *J Allergy Clin Immunol.* **105**(2 (Pt 1)):224-31.

Weinmayr, G., Weiland, S.K., Bjorksten, B. et al.(2007). Atopic Sensitization and the International Variation of Asthma Symptom Prevalence in Children.*Am. J. Respir. Crit. Care Med.* **176**(6):565-574.

WHO. Asthma Fact-sheet. Geneva: World Health Organization, 2008.

Wjs,t M, Boakye, D. (2007). Asthma in Africa. *PLoS Medicine.* **4**(2):e72.

Woodcock ,A., Addo-Yobo, E.O.D., Taggart, S.C.O., Craven. M., Custovic, A. (2001). Pet allergen levels in homes in Ghana and the United Kingdom. *The Journal of allergy and clinical immunology.* **108**(3):463-465.

Wright, R.J., Subramanian. S.V. (2007). Advancing a Multilevel Framework for Epidemiologic Research on Asthma Disparities*. *Chest.* **132**(5 suppl):757S-769S.

Yang, I., Fong, K., Holgate, S., Holloway, J. (2006.). The role of Toll-like receptors and related receptors of the innate immune system in asthma. *Curr Opin Allergy Clin Immunol.* **6**(1):23-8.

Yazdanbakhsh, M., Kremsner, P.G., van Ree. R. (2002). Allergy, Parasites, and the Hygiene Hypothesis. *Science.* **296**(5567):490-494.

Yazdanbakhsh, M., van den Biggelaar, A. and Maizels, R. M.. (2001). Th2 responses without atopy: immunoregulation in chronic helminth infections and reduced allergic disease. *Trends Immunol .* **22**(7):372-7.

Chapter 6

Mental health research in Ghana: a literature review[2]

Ursula M. Read and Victor C. Doku

Introduction

Psychiatry in Ghana is neglected in health care and research. In 1972 Adomakoh stated that 'There is a dearth of detailed knowledge of psychiatric illness in this country'(Adomakoh, 1972a). Nearly 40 years later the research record has expanded, but accurate data on epidemiology, treatment and outcomes are still sorely needed. In the absence of reliable evidence, the gaps are filled by data extrapolated from international research, "guesstimates", and anecdotal evidence. The first study of mental illness in the then Gold Coast was commissioned by the Colonial Office to study 'the forms of neurosis and psychosis among West Africans'. Tooth, a British psychiatrist, identified 400 cases of mental disorder with the help of census enumerators and chiefs (Tooth, 1950). This was followed in the 1950s by ethnographic research of people with mental disorder attending rural shrines by the British psychiatrist and anthropologist, Field (Field, 1960). The advent of the first African psychiatrist, E.B. Forster, following independence and the training of Ghanaian psychiatrists led to publication of the first clinically-based research by local psychiatrists. However, with limited resources and research expertise, the studies were small and output was limited.

This situation has persisted until recently. The majority of research in mental health has been undertaken by the country's few hard-pressed psychiatrists, occasionally assisted by expatriate researchers or clinicians, and has remained small in scale. However, recently a new impetus for mental health in Ghana has seen the establishment of mental health NGOs, the drafting of a new mental health bill, increased training for psychiatrists and psychiatric nurses, proposals for training new cadres of primary health care specialists in mental health, and increased media attention. Alongside these developments has been an increase in

---

2   Previously published as Read, U.M and Doku, V.D (2012).Mental Health Research in Ghana: a literature review. Ghana *Medical Journal*, 46(2),29-38.

the number of research projects and publications on mental health from diverse of disciplines including psychology, sociology and anthropology. A mental health research team at Kintampo Health Research Centre has conducted studies of risk factors for psychosis, mental disorders among older people, and an ethnography of psychosis (Read et al., 2009; Read, forthcoming), and an epidemiology of postnatal depression. The Mental Health and Poverty Project, which conducted research on mental health policy in four African countries including Ghana (Flisher et al., 2007), last year produced several publications in indexed journals (Ae-Ngibise et al., 2010; Akpalu et al., 2010; Awenva et al., 2010; Ofori-Atta et al., 2010a; Ofori-Atta et al., 2010b). The PubMed indexing of the *African Journal of Psychiatry* and the online publication of the *Ghana Medical Journal* (GMJ) present new opportunities for mental health research in Ghana to provide a much-needed contribution to the research record on African mental health regionally and internationally.

This paper aims to provide an overview of the current state of research on mental health in Ghana, and a critical review of published research papers. We also aim to synthesise the findings and opinions of these papers to make suggestions for priority areas for mental health research in Ghana which we hope will be of value to both clinicians and researchers in the field.

Methods

A literature search was conducted of social science and medical journals in Ghana and the UK. The authors conducted an on-line search of Pubmed using MeSH terms '*psychiatry AND Ghana*', '*mental disorders AND Ghana*', '*mental health services AND Ghana*', '*mental health AND Ghana*', '*self-injurious behaviour AND Ghana*', in addition to a manual search of the libraries of Korle-Bu Teaching Hospital (KBTH), the Institute of Psychiatry, UK, and the London School of Hygiene and Tropical Medicine (LSHTM). Ninety nine articles published between 1955-2009 were identified. Thity three articles were excluded (see Table 1). Sixty-six were included in this review. Articles were grouped under the most relevant topics, but there was overlap in some papers (see Table 2).

Table 6.1: Excluded papers from Mental Health in Ghana Search

Reason for exclusion	Number	Author/date
Unavailable	13	Addo-Kufuor and Osei, 1993; Asare and Koranteng, 1996; Lamptey, 1980; Lamptey, 1996; Lamptey, 2000; Lamptey, 2001a; Lamptey, 2001b; Osei, 2004; Turkson, 1996; Turkson and Dua, 1996; Danquah, 1979; Lamptey, 1981; Agbleze, 1970.
Opinion piece/obituary	6	Adomakoh, 1972a; Asare, 2001; Ewusi-Mensah, 2001; Margetts,1972; Roberts, 2001; Rosenberg, 2002.
Specialised case studies	3	Lamptey, 1972; Turkson and Asamoah, 1999; Turkson, 1996.
Obsolete treatment methods/ diagnosis	3	Adomakoh, 1973; Forster, 1965; Johnson and Majodina, 1979.
Neuropsychiatric effects of physical conditions	2	Dugbartey, Dugbartey and Apedo, 1998; Asare, 1996.
Specialist subfield – mental retardation, older people	3	de Graft-Johnson, 1964; Turkson, 1997; Walker, 1982.
Epilepsy	3	Adomakoh 1972b; Johnson 1980; Turkson 1990
Total	**33**	

Table 6.2: Reviewed Papers on Mental Health in Ghana by topic

Psychiatric hospital studies	5	Adomakoh, 1972; Forster, 1966; Forster, 1968; Lamptey, 1977; Turkson and Asante, 1997.
General hospital studies	2	Lamptey, 1978; Turkson, 1998.
Community studies	2	Field, 1958; Osei, 2003.
Psychosis/schizophrenia	4	Field, 1968; Fortes and Mayer, 1966; Turkson, 2000; Sikanartey and Eaton, 1984.
Depression	5	Dorahy et al., 2000; Field, 1955; Majodina and Johnson, 1983; Osei, 2001; Turkson and Dua, 1996
Suicide and self-harm	5	Adomakoh, 1975; Eshun, 2000; Eshun, 2003; Hjelmeland et al., 2008; Roberts and Nkum, 1989.
Substance misuse/alcoholism	8	Affinnih, 1999a; Affinnih, 1999b; Akyeampong, 1995; Amarquaye, 1967; Lamptey, 2005; Ofori-Akyeah and Lewis, 1972; Redvers et al., 2006; Turkson et al., 1996.
Women's mental health	5	Avotri and Walters, 1999; Avotri and Walters, 2001; Bennett et al., 2004; Turkson, 1992; Weobong et al., 2009.
Clinical picture/case studies	6	Forster, 1970; Forster, 1972a; Forster and Danquah, 1977; Osei, 2003; Turkson, 1998.
Psychopharmacy	3	Adomakoh, 1972; Mensah and Yeboah, 2003; Sanati, 2009.

Help-seeking/family response	6	Appiah-Poku et al., 2004; Fosu, 1981; Fosu, 1995; Ofori-Atta and Linden, 1995: Quinn, 2007; Read et al., 2009.
Traditional healers	4	Brautigam and Osei, 1979; Osei, 2001; Twumasi, 1972; Yeboah, 1994
Mental health services and policy	7	Ferri et al., 2004; Flisher et al., 2007; Forster, 1962a; Forster,1971; Laugharne and Burns, 1999; Laugharne et a.,l 2009; Osei, 1993.
Psychological interventions	1	Gilbert, 2005.
Review/history	2	Forster,1962b; Forste,1972b.
Poverty	1	De-Graft Aikins and Ofori-Atta, 2007.
TOTAL	**66**	

Results

Epidemiology

Early researchers and clinicians commonly predicted an increase in mental disorders in Ghana as a result of the presumed stresses of industrialisation and 'acculturation' (Field, 1958; Forster, 1970). Yet, to date, the true prevalence of mental illness in Ghana remains uncertain. Epidemiological studies are characterised by small numbers and rely on clinical case-finding methods. Prevalence rates drawn from such data are below what would be expected from international comparative studies and, in the absence of data from population-based epidemiological studies, are likely to be an underestimation.

Since psychiatric hospitals are the most easily accessible research sites, particularly for hard-pressed clinicians, a number of studies have been undertaken drawing on records at the Accra Psychiatric Hospital (APH). In a study of first admissions to APH between 1951 and 1971, Forster observed a sharp increase in admissions from 265 in 1951 to 2,284 in 1967 followed by a decline to 736 in 1971 (Forster, 1972). He attributed this to the political crisis between 1961-1966. However, since then, admissions approximate the 1960s figure despite political stability and economic development in recent years. Hospital admissions are unreliable indicators of psychiatric morbidity since they are confounded by population growth and increased awareness and exclude many cases who do not attend psychiatric services (Ferri et al, 2004).

The few community-based prevalence studies do not employ standardised research diagnoses or epidemiological methods (Field, 1958; Sikanartey and

Eaton, 1984; Fortes and Mayer, 1966; Osei, 2003). In Kumasi 194 participants were interviewed using the mental state examination (MSE) and the Self-Reporting Questionnaire (SRQ). 38 were diagnosed with depressive illness, of which 33 were women. Five women were diagnosed with schizophrenia and five men with somatisation disorder. Despite the limitations of the methodology, the author calculated an overall prevalence of psychiatric illness of 27.51 percent (Osei, 2003). Noting the popularity of prayer camps and shrines in the treatment of mental disorders, Turkson (2000) suggests that epidemiological studies of mental illness in Ghana should include thesecamps and shrines.

Schizophrenia/psychosis

In 1968, Field stated there had been an explosive increase in schizophrenia within the last 20 years (Field, 1968; p.31). However, she had no data with which to substantiate such a claim. Her longitudinal study of hundreds of cases attending rural shrines in Ashanti and Brong Ahafo regions provided a wealth of clinical and contextual detail, though she did not quantify most of her work (Field, 1955, 1958, 1968). In one exception, she approached chiefs and elders of rural towns and villages and identified 41 cases of chronic schizophrenia in 12 villages with a combined population of 4,283. In the 1960s, Fortes and Mayer, an anthropologist and his wife, a medical doctor, conducted a study of psychosis among the Tallensi in northern Ghana. Mayer diagnosed 17 cases of psychosis, 8 men and 9 women (Fortes and Mayer, 1966). Both Tooth and Field acknowledged the limitations of their methodology which relied on the assistance of chiefs and community elders.

In the 1980s, a study of the prevalence of schizophrenia in Labadi, Greater Accra, using clinical interviews and a review of medical records identified 28 cases of schizophrenia including 19 males in a population of 45,195. Thity one vagrants were also found to be psychotic (Sikanartey and Eaton, 1984). The authors restricted their methods to tracing cases from APH and Pantang Hospital, screening patients at the polyclinic, visiting a shrine and assessing 175 vagrants. No house-to-house case-finding was conducted.

Studies at APH consistently record schizophrenia and psychosis as the most commonly recorded diagnosis for about 70-75 percent of inpatients (Adomakoh, 1972a; Forster, 1962). In the only identified study of offenders with mental disorders at APH, most had been diagnosed with psychotic illness including 31 percent with schizophrenia, 20.2 percent with drug-induced psychoses, and 13.3 percent with non-specified psychosis. Most of those charged with murder or attempted murder had been diagnosed with psychotic illness, nearly half (48.6 percent) with schizophrenia (Turkson and Asante, 1997). The preponderance of schizophrenia as a diagnosis among inpatients continues to the present day. This is probably because only the most severe cases are admitted. The symptoms of acute psychosis also present grave difficulties for family members to manage at home, and are likely to prompt help-seeking. A Delphi consensus study of resource utilisation for neuropsychiatric disorders in developing countries, including Ghana, suggested that acute psychosis, manic episodes, and severe depression were the most common disorders treated within inpatient psychiatric care (Ferri et al., 2004).

Depression

Colonial psychiatrists commonly asserted the virtual absence of depression among Africans, which was later challenged by Field, among others. Field surmised that the self-accusations of women who confessed to witchcraft were akin to the self-reproach expressed by women with depression in Britain (Field, 1955, 1960). She observed that 'depression is the commonest mental illness of Akan rural women' (1960: 149). Two studies of psychiatric morbidity in general hospitals and clinics suggest that more neurotic and affective disorders may be seen in these facilities than in the psychiatric hospitals although numbers are small (Lamptey, 1978; Turkson, 1998). In a survey of psychiatric morbidity at six polyclinics in Accra, of 172 patients, 27 were found to have psychiatric illness, with a further 7 having physical illness with concomitant psychiatric illness. Of these 23 (72 percent) were diagnosed with 'neurosis' (Lamptey, 1978). Although Lamptey recorded no cases of depression, however, it is possible these may have been missed due to the prominence of somatic symptoms such as palpitations, burning sensations and insomnia. In another study of 94 patients referred to a psychiatric outpatient clinic at KBTH, the majority were diagnosed with affective (23) and neurotic/stress-related disorders (11) (Turkson, 1998).

To address the lack of cross-cultural data on depression in the early 1980s , the World Health Organization sponsored a study utilising the Standardized Assessment for Depressive Disorders (SADD). Fifty patients were assessed using SADD, 33 were female. Anxiety and tension were the core symptoms expressed by participants, with 35 percent reporting feelings of guilt and self-reproach. Feelings of sadness and loss of interest and enjoyment were commonly reported. Forty reported somatic symptoms including headaches, bodily heat, and generalised body pain (Majodina and Johnson, 1983). The authors argue that there has been a change in the presentation of depression in Africa compared to earlier data. However, whilst the population of Ghana is more widely educated than in the 1950s, the study recruited a highly selective English-speaking sample who had already interpreted their symptoms in such as way as to approach psychiatric hospital.

Indeed, Turkson and Dua's study with a larger, less well-educated sample produced contrasting results. They studied 131 female outpatients with a diagnosis of depression using the Montgomery-Asberg Depressive Rating Scale (MADRS). They noted a high degree of somatic symptoms, in particular headaches (77.86 percent) and sleeplessness (68.7 percent). In contrast to the SADD study, there were fewer reported psychological symptoms such as pessimistic thoughts (20.61 percent) and sadness (12.97 percent). Only 10 (7.3 percent) reported suicidal thoughts (Turkson and Dua, 1996). However the MADRS has fewer psychological items than the SADD and therefore elicits different symptoms, highlighting one of the limitations of standardised instruments, particularly where they have not been validated with the local population.

Osei explored the incidence of depression among 17 self-confessed 'witches' at three shrines in the Ashanti Region of Ghana. All were diagnosed with depression according to International Classification of Diseases (ICD-10). Three also had serious physical health problems. As in the previous studies, many described physical complaints such as a burning sensation or persistent headaches. The women also expressed ideas of guilt relating to having harmed someone in the family through the use of witchcraft (Osei, 2001). Like Field, Osei suggests that guilt feelings arising from depression might prompt women to confess to witchcraft. Such research raises interesting issues for the study of mental illness within the context of widespread belief in witchcraft and other supernatural phenomena in Ghana.

Turkson and Dua (1996) hypothesise on a link between socio-economic status and depression, but without a control group and with inadequate numbers, they provide little substantive evidence. A qualitative study of 75 women in the Volta Region is highly suggestive of a link between social factors and psychological distress (Walters et al., 2003; Avotri and Walters, 1999; Avotri and Walters, 2001). While this study did not set out specifically to research mental disorders, almost three-quarters of the women interviewed described 'thinking too much' or 'worrying too much'. Importantly, such symptoms were more prominent in women's accounts of their health than physical health problems. Most participants complained of stresses arising from multiple responsibilities in the arenas of family and work, as well as financial hardship (Avotri and Walters, 1999). Headaches, bodily aches and pains, and sleep disturbance were commonly reported. A similar link between such experiences of poverty and possible symptoms of mental illness such as excessive thinking, worry and anxiety, as well as persistent physical symptoms such as headaches, has been made in a study of vagrants and squatters in Accra (de-Graft Aikins and Ofori-Atta, 2007). It is probable that some of these women may have met the criteria for a psychiatric diagnosis of depression.

The prominence of somatic symptoms among Ghanaian women diagnosed with depression is notable. Turkson (1998) notes that in 1988 32 percent of all new patients at APH presented with primarily somatic symptoms such as headaches, burning sensations, tiredness and bodily weakness, with the majority diagnosed with anxiety, depression and somatisation disorders. This highlights the importance of screening measures which have been locally validated and can identify somatic and non-somatic symptoms. A study of depression and life satisfaction among Nigerian, Australian, Northern Irish, Swazi and Ghanaian college students utilising the Beck Depression Inventory (BDI) for example, found that Ghanaians had significantly lower depression scores than other groups (Dorahy et al., 2000). Aside from sleeplessness and loss of appetite, the BDI items are mostly concerned with psychological aspects of depression such as worthlessness and guilt. In a study of the comparative validity of screening scales for post-natal common mental disorders, Weobong provides evidence for the cross-cultural validity and reliability of a Twi version of the Patient Health Questionnaire (PHQ-9) (Weobong et al., 2009). Significantly, the study showed that a mixture of somatic and cognitive symptoms discriminated best between cases and non-cases for all scales evaluated.

Given the high birth rate in Ghana, Weobong's study of post-natal depression will provide much-needed data on a condition which has been little researched. The only previous study identified described four cases of psychiatric disorders associated with childbirth treated at APH, including post-partum psychosis and manic-depressive psychosis. The author observed that few cases were referred to the psychiatric hospital and queried whether post-partum mental disorders were being recognised within antenatal wards. He also noted the influence of social factors such as marital problems and financial difficulties (Turkson, 1992).

The literature reveals that women are generally under-represented in psychiatric hospitals in Ghana. In Forster's (1972) study of APH inpatient admissions between 1951-1971, males consistently outnumbered females by about 3:1. It has been suggested that when men become acutely mentally unwell, they may be more difficult to manage at home, and so are more likely to be brought to the psychiatric hospitals for treatment (Sikanartey and Eaton, 1984; Osei, 2001, 2003; Jahoda, 1979). Women in Ghana appear to be underserved by mental health services and the majority of women suffering from mental disorders, particularly depression, remain untreated or under the care of churches and shrines. Research at facilities such as polyclinics, shrines and churches may provide a more accurate picture of the numbers of women with mental disorders and their clinical presentation.

Suicide and self-harm

There is very little research on self-harm in Ghana. Roberts and Nkum (1989) examined the case notes of 53 patients admitted to Komfo Anokye Teaching Hospital (KATH) over a five-year period. The most common means of self-harm was ingestion of pesticides (22), and other harmful substances. 10 used 'physical methods' including self-stabbing (4). Six cases were diagnosed with psychosis and 28 with acute reactions to social stresses such as marital and financial problems. The authors found an increase in deliberate self-harm during the five-year period of their study compared to an earlier study from 0.3 cases per 1,000 admissions between 1965-1971 to 1.32 cases per 1,000 admissions in 1987 (Adomakoh, 1975). Based on their findings, the authors estimated a crude annual incidence of 2.93 per 100,000. However, this figure is likely to be an underestimate given that some cases may not reach medical services.

A number of studies comparing suicidal ideation among Ghanaian and Caucasian students in the USA showed significantly lower rates of self-reported suicidal ideation among the Ghanaian sample, as well as more negative attitudes towards suicide (Eshun, 2000; Eshun, 2003). A larger survey compared 570 Ghanaian students with students from Uganda and Norway utilising the Attitudes Toward Suicide Questionnaire. Thirty (5.4 percent) of the Ghanaian sample reported making suicide attempts, significantly lower than either Uganda or Norway. 53 reported suicide attempts in their(?) family, and 192 amongst other families (?). Nine reported a completed suicide in the family, and

91 among non-family members, again markedly lower than those reported by the Ugandan and Norwegian respondents (Hjelmeland et al., 2008).

Although these studies seem to suggest a low rate of suicidal ideation in Ghana, generalisation is cautioned since all the studies were conducted with young, urbanised, highly educated participants. There is also no published research on completed suicides in Ghana. It is possible that the lower reported rates of suicidal ideation or suicide attempts may in part reflect a likelihood that Ghanaian students would be less likely to report suicidal ideation due to negative attitudes towards suicide. This is supported by the finding of Hjelmeland et al., (2008) that 31 percent of their sample felt that suicide should not be talked about. However, these studies also point to possible factors in Ghanaian society which could be employed in suicide prevention including family support, religious belief, and an emphasis on the value of the group. Qualitative studies related to beliefs and attitudes towards suicide, as well as risk factors, would greatly enhance the quantitative data and enable an exploration of some of the correlations observed (Eshun, 2003).

There is one recent study on anorexia nervosa among female secondary school students in North East Ghana, a condition which has been considered rare in non-Western cultures (Bennet et al, 2004). The researchers completed a clinical examination of physical and mental health, two standard measures of eating behaviour and attitudes, and a depression screen. Of 666 students, 29 were pathologically underweight, among whom 10 were diagnosed with morbid self-starvation based on clinically significant indicators such as denial of hunger, self-punishment and perfectionist traits. The majority of the participants, both Christian and Muslim, reported regularly engaging in religious fasting. For the 10 engaged in morbid self-starvation, this fasting was particularly frequent, at least once a week, and associated with feelings of self-control and self-punishment. Since self-starvation was not associated with a desire to be thin nor a morbid fear of fatness, a diagnosis of anorexia nervosa according to DSM-IV or ICD-10 criteria could not be made. However, the authors suggest that in Ghana, fasting rather than dieting may provide the cultural context within which morbid self-starvation occurs (Bennet et al., 2004). As suggested by the role of somatic symptoms in the presentation of depression in Ghana, this study has important implications regarding the limitations of standardised psychiatric diagnoses and the need to recognise cultural influences on the presentation of mental illness. Further research could help to develop more culturally sensitive diagnostic criteria and screening tools.

Substance misuse

It is notable that the highest number of published papers in this review concerns substance abuse (Akyeampong, 1995; Affinih, 1999a, 1999b; Amarquaye, 1967; Danquah, 1979; Lamptey, 1996, 2001, 2005; Ofori-Akyeah and Lewis, 1972; Redvers et al., 2006). This may reflect more the interests of researchers than the severity of the problem. In his sociological study, Affinnih claims there has been an increase in the use of drugs such as cocaine and heroin in Accra and other urban centres (Affinih, 1999a, 1999b). However, data from the psychiatric hospitals suggest that cannabis and alcohol are the most frequently used substances and may be a risk factor for the development of psychosis among young men (Foster, 1966; Turkson and Asante, 1997; Turkson, 1988; Redvers et al., 2006).

However, there is limited research on the mental health implications of substance use in Ghana. A study of substance abusers admitted to a private clinic in Accra excluded those with co-morbid mental illness (Lamptey, 2005). Importantly only two papers were identified which were primarily concerned with alcohol misuse, one of which is a social history of alcohol use in Ghana (Akyeampong, 1995). The only epidemiological study of alcohol misuse was conducted with 350 psychiatric outpatients in Kumasi using the WHO Alcohol Use Disorders Identification Test (AUDIT). The researchers found a prevalence of only 8.6 percent for hazardous drinking, significantly lower than comparable studies in the West (Redvers et al., 2006). The link between substance misuse and mental disorders may be exaggerated in the public imagination and the media and there is a tendency to make speculative assertions based on limited evidence. Affinnih (1999a) for example quotes a minister of health as saying that 'drugs are responsible for 70 percent of the cases in local psychiatric hospitals' (p.397), a figure which is not substantiated by hospital records. More research is needed in this area from a specifically mental health perspective.

Help-seeking

The popularity of traditional healers in the treatment of mental illness has been noted since the earliest studies of mental illness in Ghana and continues to the present day (Laugharne and Burns, 1999). A study of 194 people attending three shrines in the Ashanti Region stated that 100 (51.55 percent) of these were suffering from a mental illness, the majority (64 or 32.99 percent)) with depression. Another 14 were diagnosed with somatisation, and 19 with psychotic illness, including 6 with schizophrenia, 4 with acute psychosis and 3 with cannabis-induced psychosis (Osei, 2001a, 2001b).

Though data are limited, two papers suggest a change in the pattern of help-seeking over the last 30 years, with a greater role for Christian healers. In 1973, a study of 105 patients at APH diagnosed with psychosis showed that almost all (97 or 92 percent)) had sought another form of treatment before attending the psychiatric hospital. 67 (64 percent) patients had consulted a herbalist, 28 (26 percent) a healing church, and only 2 a fetish priest (Lamptey, 1977). A study in 2004 of the use of traditional healers and pastors by 303 new patients attending state and private psychiatric services in Kumasi found that a smaller proportion of patients had consulted other forms of treatment and a greater number reported consulting a pastor rather than a traditional healer (43 or 14.2 percent, and 18 or 5.9 percent respectively). There also appeared to be more use of medical facilities in the treatment of mental illness. Fourteen patients had seen a family doctor and 6 had visited another psychiatric hospital. Nearly a quarter (24.4 percent) had previously attended one of the other mental health centres in Kumasi (Appiah-Poku et al., 2004).

Since the early ethnographic studies, little research has been conducted on beliefs and attitudes towards mental illness in Ghana which may influence help-seeking behaviour, though there is much speculation on the spiritual attribution of mental illness among the general population (Ae-Ngibise et al., 2010). Two studies conducted in the early 1990s suggest a more varied and complex picture. A quantitative survey of 1,000 women in Accra found that most (88 percent) said they would seek help from the psychiatric hospitals and only a minority (8.2 percent) said they would consult traditional healers. The most important socio-demographic factors influencing the orientation towards help-seeking were area of residence, ethnicity, migration status, and prior use of medical services. Women who perceived the cause of psychosis to be natural or stress-related were more likely to seek help from mental hospitals than those who identified supernatural causation (Fosu, 1995).

Similarly, a study of the effect of social change on causal beliefs of mental disorders and treatment preferences among teachers in Accra found that rather than emphasising spiritual causation for mental illness in Ghana, respondents attributed multiple causal factors to mental illness drawn from biological, social and spiritual models (Ofori-Atta and Linden, 1995). The authors attributed this in part to 'acculturation' but cautioned that participants may have wished to present themselves as educated and therefore would have been less willing to disclose supernatural beliefs. They also hypothesised that such beliefs may only come into play as an 'indirect attribution' (Ofori-Atta and Linden 1995).

In both studies, participants were urban residents and most were educated. It is possible that research with a rural and less educated sample would yield different results as a more recent qualitative study has suggested. Using semi-structured interviews with 80 relatives of people with mental illness, and 10 service providers, Quinn (2007) explored beliefs about mental illness in Accra and Kumasi, and two rural areas in the Ashanti and Northern regions and how these influenced family responses to mental illness. In common with the earlier studies which suggested a process of 'acculturation' among urban residents (Tooth, 1950; Fortes and Mayer, 1966), Quinn reported that in urban areas most respondents attributed mental illness to 'natural' causes such as work stress. In the Northern Region, however, spiritual attribution was more common. The Northern sample were also significantly less educated, with 14 out of 19 respondents having no education. Caution should be exercised in generalising these results as the sample size in each area was small. There were also many 'don't knows' – 22 out of 80 (Quinn, 2007). This may be a reflection of more complex aetiological beliefs and uncertainty about the cause of mental illness than reflected in a binary spiritual/natural schema, as earlier studies have suggested (Jahoda, 1979; Ofori-Atta and Linden, 1995).

Quinn's study claims that there was greater reliance on traditional healing in the north due to beliefs in a spiritual origin of mental illness, however it does not explore these issues in sufficient depth to support this assertion. The lower education of those in the Northern sample as well as their long distance from the psychiatric hospitals were other factors which may have influenced help-seeking. The study also reports that respondents in the Northern Region described greater acceptance of people with mental illness by families and communities, with little evidence of stigma, echoing earlier reports (Tooth, 1950; Fortes and Mayer, 1966). Quinn's (2007) finding however is based on only 19 respondents, 17 of whom were male. Since mothers are likely to provide most of the caring, they might have provided differing opinions on the impact of the illness.

None of these studies allow for in-depth exploration of possible influences on help-seeking behaviour for mental illness. However, they suggest some interesting hypotheses regarding the reputation of traditional healers in treating mental illness, the stigma attached to mental illness and psychiatric hospitals, and the scarcity of psychiatric services. This points to important lines for future qualitative research, including some using anthropological/ethnographic methodologies.

In common with other mental health researchers and professionals in Africa, the authors of these studies recommend collaboration with traditional and faith healers in the treatment of mental illness, such as training healers in recognising severe mental illness, and referring patients to psychiatric services. However, traditional healers and pastors may be unwilling to pass on their customers to biomedical practitioners or admit to failings in their intervention. Claims for the efficacy of traditional healers also tend to be anecdotal and speculative and are seldom based on rigorous longitudinal data. Most authors highlight the role of traditional healers in addressing the psychosocial aspects of mental illness and their resonance with cultural beliefs (Jahoda, 1979; Lamptey, 1977; Brautigam and Osei, 1979; Roberts, 2001; Ewusi-Mensah, 2001). While some present a rather idealised picture (Brautigam and Osei, 1979), others note the inhumane treatment of people with mental illness by traditional healers (Read et al., 2009; Osei, 2001b; Roberts, 2001). One paper points to the role of the family in caring for patients within traditional shrines and churches, and shows how this model was replicated within psychiatric facilities by enabling family members to stay with the patient in hospital (Osei, 1993). Further research is needed on the practices of traditional and faith healers to inform interventions that reduce the maltreatment of people with mental illness, and ensure that those with mental illness receive the best quality treatment from both psychiatric facilities and informal services.

Discussion

This review shows that mental health research in Ghana remains limited in both quantity and quality. In the absence of a comprehensive research record, much is assumed based on scant evidence, and services are heavily influenced by the results of research conducted elsewhere, most often in high-income settings. While researchers have used their findings to argue for more resources for mental health, such pleas would be more forcefully made were there more accurate epidemiological data. It is difficult to estimate the true prevalence of mental disorder and plan effectively for mental health promotion and treatment without more rigorous, large-scale population-based studies. However, the published research on mental disorders such as psychosis, depression, substance abuse and self-harm provides glimpses into promising future avenues for exploration of the cultural context of these disorders in Ghana, including risk factors, with important implications for clinical intervention and mental health promotion.

A major omission in the literature is studies of the practice and efficacy of psychiatric treatment in Ghana. Given the scarcity of psychosocial interventions, psychotropic medication is the mainstay of treatment and is the topic of four papers (Sanati, 2009; Adomakoh, 1972b; Forster 1965; Mensah and Yeboah, 2003). One study reports that adherence to medication is poor among many patients, suggesting the need for further research into the reasons for this, and methods for improving both access and adherence (Mensah and Yeboah, 2003). Most research in Ghana has been conducted by psychiatrists and there is very little published research by psychologists, psychiatric nurses and social workers. The only published study identified on counselling argued for consideration of notions of self-identity, as well as the influence of the multi-lingual post-colonial environment when importing talking therapies (Gilbert, 2006), a topic which would benefit from further research. Multidisciplinary research is also needed on the particular social and psychological factors which play an important part in the aetiology and course of mental disorders within Ghana and how these might be addressed.

Research on beliefs and attitudes towards mental illness suggests that these influence not only help-seeking behaviour but also stigma, care-giving and social inclusion. Research in this area may not only point to the roots of stigma, social exclusion and human rights abuse, but also to potential resources for the support and social integration of those with mental disorders. Most importantly, research on mental health in Ghana needs to listen to the voices of those who live with mental disorders, and those who care for them. Existing research suggests a high social, financial and psychological burden for patients and care givers (Read et al., 2009; Avotri and Walters, 1999, 2001; Quinn, 2007), and further research in this area could provide a powerful tool to argue for greater attention to mental illness as vital but neglected public health concern.

Conclusion

The studies reviewed in this paper have been generally small in scale and and, therefore, inappropriate for generalization. Nonetheless, they provide important insights into the development of mental health care in Ghana and the clinical picture, and suggest directions for future research. Based on this review, we suggest the following priorities for mental health research in Ghana:

1. Epidemiological studies of mental disorders – these should be population-based to capture as many cases as possible, and include shrines and churches.
2. Research on mental disorders, in particular psychosis, substance use, depression, somatisation, and self-harm including risk factors, clinical picture, course and outcome.
3. Outcome studies of interventions within psychiatric services, primary care and other service providers e.g. NGOs.
4. The experiences of people with mental illness and their family members, including the psychosocial and financial impact, help-seeking and experiences of treatment.
5. The practices of traditional and religious healers and potential for collaboration.

Evidently, these topics call for both quantitative and qualitative methodologies across disciplines in both medicine and social science. However an important caveat concerns who will conduct this research, given the pressures on clinicians and the limited research expertise. For too long, mental health research has been dominated by experts in high-income countries, with the consequent risk of cultural bias, underscoring the need for research in Africa by Africans. There remains a need for capacity building among clinicians across all disciplines to conduct clinically-based research, and for researchers trained in psychiatric epidemiological methods. Collaboration with mental health researchers in Africa and elsewhere, including the Ghanaian diaspora, is one suggestion (Doku and Mallett, 2003). Above all, high-quality large-scale research requires funding. Given the burden of mental illness suggested by existing research in Ghana and elsewhere in the region, there is a strong case for international funding for mental health research to provide an evidence-based foundation for targeted and culturally relevant interventions.

References

Adomakoh, C.C. (1972a) Mental hospital patients: A Castle Road profile. *Ghana Med. J.* 1972;2:65-71.

Adomakoh, C.C. (1972b) Prevalence of motor disorders in Phenothiazine treated psychotics in mental hospital. *Ghana Med. J.* 1972:149-53.

Adomakoh, C.C. (1975). A preliminary report on attempted suicides seen in a general hospital in Ghana. *Ghana Med. J.* 14:323-236.

Ae-Ngibise, K., Cooper, S., Adiibokah, E., Akpalu, B., Lund. C., Doku, V. (2010).'Whether you like it or not people with mental problems are going to go to them': A qualitative exploration into the widespread use of traditional and faith healers in the provision of mental health care in Ghana. *International Review of Psychiatry* . 22(6):558-67.

Affinnih, Y.H. (1999a). A preliminary study of drug abuse and its mental health and health consequences among addicts in Greater Accra, Ghana. *J. Psychoactive Drugs* 1999;31(4):395-403.

Affinnih, Y,H. (1999b). Drug use in greater Accra, Ghana: pilot study. *Subst. Use Misuse* 1999;34(2):157-69.

Akpalu, B,, Lund, C,, Doku, V,, Ofori-Att,a A,. Osei, A., Ae-Ngibise, K. et al. (2010). Scaling up community-based services and improving quality of care in the state psychiatric hospitals: the way forward for Ghana *African Journal of Psychiatry.* 13:109-15.

Akyeampong ,E. (1995).Alcoholism in Ghana: A socio-cultural exploration. *Culture Medicine and Psychiatry.*19(2):261-80.

Amarquaye, F.K. (1967). Indian hemp ingestion in Ghana. *Ghana Med. J.* 6(6):126-30.

Appiah-Poku, J., Laugharn.e R., Mensah. E., Osei. Y., Burns,T. (2004). Previous help sought by patients presenting to mental health services in Kumasi, Ghana. *Soc. Psychiatry Psychiatr. Epidemiol.* 39:208-11.

Avotri, J.Y. and Walters, V. (1999). "You just look at our work and see if you have any freedom on earth": Ghanaian women's accounts of their work and their health. *Soc. Sci. Med.* 48:1123-33.

Avotri, J.Y., Walters, V. (2001). "We women worry a lot about our husbands": Ghanaian women talking about their health and their relationships with men. *Journal of Gender Studies.* 10(2):197-211.

Awenva, D., Read. U.M., Ofori-Attah, A,L,, Doku, V.C.K., Osei, A.O., Flisher, A.J. et al. (2010). From mental health policy development in Ghana to implementation: What are the barriers? *African Journal of Psychiatry.* 13:184-91.

Bennett, D., Sharpe, M., Freeman, C., Carson, A. (2004).Anorexia nervosa among female secondary school students in Ghana. *Br. J. Psychiatry.* 185:312-7.

Brautigam, W. and Osei. Y. (1978). Psychosomatic Illness Concept Among the Akan of Ghana. *Canadian Journal of Psychiatry.* 24:451-57.

Danquah, S.A. (1979). Drug abuse among Ghanaian students. *Psychopathologie Africaine* 15:201-11.

de-Graft Aikins, A., Ofori-Atta, A.L. (2007). Homelessness and mental health in Ghana: Everyday experiences of Accra's migrant squatters. *J Health Psychol.* 12(5):761-78.

Doku, V.C.K., Mallett, M.R. (2003).Collaborating with developing countries in psychiatric research. *Br. J. Psychiatry* . 182(3):188-89.

Dorahy, M.J., Lewis, C.A., Schumaker. J.F., Akuamoah-Boateng. R., Duze, M.C., Sibiya, T,E. (2000). Depression and life satisfaction among Australian, .Ghanaian, Nigerian, Northern Irish, and Swazi university students *Journal of Social Behavior and Personality.* 15(4):569–80.

Eshun, S. (2000). Role of gender and rumination in suicide ideation: A comparison of college samples from Ghana and the United States *Cross-Cultural Research* 34(3):250-63.

Eshun, S. (2003). Sociocultural determinants of suicide ideation: a comparison between American and Ghanaian college samples. *Suicide and Life Threatening Behaviour.* 33(2):165-71.

Ewusi-Mensah, I. (2001) Post-colonial psychiatric care in Ghana. *Psychiatric Bulletin.* 25:228-29.

Ferri, C., Chisholm, D., Van Ommeren. M., Prince, M. (2004). Resource utilisation for neuropsychiatric disorders in developing countries: a multinational Delphi consensus study. *Soc. Psychiatry Psychiatr. Epidemiol.* 39(3):218-27.

Field, M. (1955). Witchcraft as a primitive interpretation of mental disorder. *Journal of Mental Science* . 101:826-33.

Field, M,J. (1958). Mental disorder in rural Ghana. *The Journal Of Mental Disease.* 1043-51.

Field, M,J. *Search for Security: An Ethno-Psychiatric Study of Rural Ghana.* London Faber and Faber 1960.

Field, M,J. (1968).Chronic psychosis in rural Ghana. *Br. J. Psychiatry.* 114:31-33.

Flisher, A.J, Lund. C., Funk, M., Banda, M., Bhana, A., Doku, V. et al. (2007). Mental health policy development and implementation in four African countries.*J Health Psychol.* 12(3):505-16.

Forster, E.B. (1962). The Theory and Practice of Psychiatry in Ghana.*Am. J. Psychother.* 16:7-51.

Forster, E.B. (1965). A study of Thioridazine Hydrochiloride on chronic schizophrenics. *Ghana Med. J.* 22-24.

Forster, E.B.F. (1966). .A longitudinal ecological study of one hundred consecutive admissions to the Accra Mental Hospital *Ghana Med. J.* 5.

Forster, E.B. (1970). Symptom formation in the African patient. *Ghana Med. J.* 201-04.

Forster, E.B. (1972). Mental health and political change in Ghana 1951-1971. *Psychopathologie Africaine.* 383-471.

Fortes, M., Mayer, D.Y. (1966). Psychosis and social change among the Tallensi of Northern Ghana. *Cahier D'Etudes Africaines.* 21:5-40.

Fosu, G.B. (1995).Women's orientation towards help-seeking for mental disorders. *Soc. Sci. Med.* 40(8):1029-40.

Gilbert J. (2006).Cultural imperialism revisited: Counselling and globalisation *International Journal of Critical Psychology.* (Special Issue: Critical Psychology in Africa, 17):10-28.

Hjelmeland, H., Akotia, C.S., Owens, V., Knizek, B.L., Nordvik, H., Schroeder, R. et al. (2008). Self-reported suicidal behavior and attitudes toward suicide and suicide prevention among psychology students in Ghana, Uganda, and Norway. *Crisis.* 29(1):20-31.

Jahoda, G. (1979). Traditional healers and other institutions concerned with mental illness in Ghana. In: Ademuwagun Z, Ayoade JA, Harrison IE, Warren DM, editors. *African Therapeutic Systems.* Waltham: African Studies Association. 98-109.

Lamptey. J.J. (1977). Patterns of Psychiatric Consultations at the Accra Psychiatric Hospital in Ghana. *African Journal of Psychiatry.* 3:123-27.

Lamptey, J.J. (1978). Psychiatric morbidity in Accra polyclinics. *Ghana Med. J.* .170-76.

Lamptey, J.J. (1996). Are opioid addicts depressed? *Ghana Med. J.* 31a:805-11.

Lamptey, J. J. (2001). Social adjustment of a group of discharged substance abusers. *Ghana Med. J.* 35:116-19.

Lamptey, J.J. (2005). Socio-demographic characteristics of substance abusers admitted to a private specialist clinic. *Ghana Med. J.* 39(1):2-7.

Laugharne, R. and Burns,T. (1999). Mental health services in Kumasi, Ghana. *Psychiatric Bulletin .* 23(6):361-63.

Majodina, M. Z., Johnson, F.Y. (1983). Standardized assessment of depressive disorders (SADD) in Ghana. *Br. J. Psychiatry .* 143:442-6.

Mensah, E.S., Yeboah, F.A. (2003). A preliminary study into the evaluation of drug compliance among psychiatric patients in Komfo Anokye Teaching Hospital, Ghana. *Ghana Med. J.* 37(2):68-71.

Ofori-Akyeah, J.and Lewis, R.A. (1972).Drug abuse among Ghanaian medical students. *Ghana Med. J.* 307.

Ofori-Atta, A.M.L.and Linden, W. (1995). The effect of social change on causal beliefs of mental disorders and treatment preferences in Ghana *Soc. Sci. Med.* 40(9):1231-42.

Ofori-Atta, A., Cooper. S,. Akpalu, B., Osei, A., Doku, V., Lund, C. et al. (2010a) Common understandings of women's mental illness in Ghana: Results from a qualitative study. *International Review of Psychiatry.* 22(6):589-98.

Ofori-Atta, A., Read, U.M., Lund, C. (2010b) A situation analysis of mental health services and legislation in Ghana: Challenges for transformation. *African Journal of Psychiatry.* 13(2):99-108.

Osei, A.O. (2001a). Witchcraft and depression: a study into the psychopathological features of alleged witches. *Ghana Med. J.* 35(3):111-15.

Osei, A.O. (2001b) Types of psychiatric illness at traditional healing centres in Ghana. *Ghana Med. J.* 35(3):106-10.

Osei, A.O (2003). Prevalence of psychiatric illness in an urban community in Ghana. *Ghana Med. J.* 37(2):62-67.

Osei, Y. (1993). Family support for psychiatric patients. *World Health Forum* 14(4):385-89.

Quinn, N. (2007). Beliefs and community responses to mental illness in Ghana: The experiences of family carers. *Int. J. Soc. Psychiatry.* 53(2):175-88.

Read, U.M. "I want the one that will heal me completely so it won't come back again": The limits of antipsychotic medication in rural Ghana. *Transcultural Psychiatry* forthcoming.

Read, U.M. (2009). Adiibokah E, Nyame S. Local suffering and the global discourse of mental health and human rights: An ethnographic study of responses to mental illness in rural Ghana. *Globalisation and Health* .5(1):13.

Redvers, A., Appiah-Poku, J., Laugharne, R. (2006). Alcohol misuse in psychiatric outpatients in Ghana. *Primary Care and Community Psychiatry.* 11:179-83.

Roberts, M.A., Nkum, B.C.(1989). Deliberate self-harm in Ghana. *Ghana Med. J.* 23(2):81-87.

Roberts, H. (2001). A way forward for mental health care in Ghana? *The Lancet* 357:1859.

Sanati, A. (2009). Investigating the quality of psychotropic drug prescriptions at Accra Psychiatric Hospital. *International Psychiatry.* 6(3):69-70.

Sikanartey, T., Eaton, W.W. (1984). Prevalence of schizophrenia in the Labadi District of Ghana. *Acta Psychiatrica Scandanavica.* 69(2):156-61.

Tooth, G. (1950). *Studies in Mental Illness in the Gold Coast.* London: H.M.S.O.,

Turkson, S.N. (1992). Psychiatric disorders associated with childbirth among Ghanaian women - illustrative cases. *Ghana Med. J.* ;26:467-70.

Turkson, S.N. (2000). Schizophrenia--the spirit possessed 23 year old male from rural Kpando Dzoanti, Volta Region in Ghana: case report. *East Afr. Med. J.* 77(11):629-30.

Turkson, S.N. (1998)> Psychiatric diagnosis among referred patients in Ghana. *East Afr. Med. J.* 75(6):336-8.

Turkson, S.N. and Dua, A.N. (1996). A study of the social and clinical characteristics of depressive illness among Ghanaian women (1988-1992). *West Afr. J. Med.* 15(2):85-90.

Turkson, S.N. and Asante, K. (1997). Psychiatric disorders among offender patients in the Accra Psychiatric Hospital. *West Afr. J. Med.* 16(2):88-92.

Walters, V., Avotri, J.Y., Charles, N. (2003). "Your heart is never free": Women in Wales and Ghana talking about distress. In: Stoppard JM, McMullen LM, editors. *Situating Sadness: Women and Depression in Social Context.* New York: New York: University Press,183-206.

Weobong, B., Akpalu, B., Doku. V., Owusu-Agyei, S., Hurt, L., Kirkwood. B, et al. (2009). The comparative validity of screening scales for postnatal common mental disorder in Kintampo, Ghana. *J. Affect. Disord.* 113(1-2):109-17.

Chapter 7

Modifiable risk factors of chronic non-communicable diseases in Ghana: insights from national and community-based surveys

Raphael Baffour Awuah and Ernest Afrifa-Anane.

Introduction

In Ghana, major causes of disability and death have shifted from predominantly communicable diseases to a combination of communicable and chronic non-communicable diseases (NCDs) over the last few decades (de-Graft-Aikins et al., 2012). The major NCDs include hypertension, stroke, diabetes and cancers.

There are a number of risk factors associated with NCDs. Some of the risk factors are non-modifiable while others are modifiable or lifestyle-based risk factors. The non-modifiable risk factors include age, gender and family history. Modifiable behavioural risk factors include tobacco use, physical inactivity, unhealthy diet and excessive alcohol.

In Ghana, there has been a rise in the prevalence of modifiable risk factors over the years. It has been suggested that urbanization, changing lifestyles (including poor diets), globalization and weak health systems are implicated in this rise (WHO, 2005; Agyei-Mensah and de-Graft Aikins, 2010).

The aim of this chapter is to provide a synthesis of the existing research on modifiable risk factors of NCDs in Ghana and to examine the implications of these risk factors for hypertension and diabetes.

Methods

We conducted a standard literature review of published empirical studies on the modifiable risk factors of hypertension and diabetes. We searched for published research on NCD risk factors in Ghana on PubMed. We also accessed grey literature, and included submitted manuscripts and Masters theses from the Regional Institute of Population Studies (RIPS). Empirical studies on NCDs in

Ghana employing quantitative methods were included in the synthesis. Most of the data derived from quantitative methods were cross sectional surveys. Some of the surveys included the Global School Health Survey, conducted in 2007, the World Health Survey, conducted in 2003 and the Ghana Demographic and Health Survey, conducted in 2008. Two rounds of the Urban Poverty and Health Survey conducted by RIPS in three poor communities in Accra were also included. The first and second waves of the Women's Health Study of Accra (WHSA-I and WHSA-II) were also included in this synthesis. The majority of studies on NCDs (particularly hypertension and diabetes) were conducted in the Greater Accra and Ashanti regions. We will present the results of our synthesis by thematic areas, namely: obesity, smoking, alcohol consumption and physical (in)activity. We also present profiles of prevalence studies in Table 7.1.

Results

Obesity

Obesity is a condition of abnormal or excessive fat accumulation in adipose tissue (Garrow, 1988). Body mass index (BMI) is used as a proxy definition of obesity and this is expressed as the ratio of one's weight (kg) and the square of height (meters), which is greater than or equal to $30kg/m^2$ (WHO, 2004). Obesity is a form of malnutrition and constitutes a major risk factor for NCDs; especially diabetes, hypertension and related heart diseases (Biritwum et al., 2005; Popkin and Gordon-Larsen, 2004).

Obesity is a growing health problem in both developed industrialized countries and developing countries (Duda et al., 2007). Isidoro et al. (2011) report that it is the second major risk factor after smoking for all-cause cancers; for instance breast cancers in post-menopausal women. Burke et al., (2005) have also argued that the increase in the prevalence of obesity and overweight implies increase in lifestyle diseases such as hypertension, Type 2 diabetes and cardiovascular diseases. The amount of calorie intake, time spent doing physical activity, time spent in sedentary occupation as well as smoking and alcohol intake have been associated with the prevalence of obesity (Biritwum et al., 2005; Addo et al., 2009).

Prevalence of obesity

Studies on the prevalence of obesity in Ghana have been conducted using both national and community-based data (Biritwum et al., 2005; Duda et al., 2007). Some studies have compared samples of Ghanaian migrants to Ghanaian residents (Agyemang et al., 2008). A few studies have been institution-based (Aryeetey and Ansong, 2011).

In Ghana, like other sub-Saharan African countries, there is a significant incidence of obesity, especially among those living in urban areas, although the situation was different about a generation ago (Amoah, 2003; Walker, 1994). Studies on the prevalence of obesity in Ghana date from 1987. A prevalence of 0.9 percent for both men and women aged 20 years and above was recorded between 1987 to 1988 (WHO TRS, 1995). By 2003, Biritwum et al. (2005) had recorded a national prevalence of 5.5 percent among the population 18 years and above. Duda et al., (2007), reporting results of the first round of the Women's Health Study of Accra conducted in 2003, indicated a prevalence of 34.7 percent for women. Amoah ,(2003) also reported a prevalence of 14.1 percent for 752 women in Accra. The Ghana Demographic and Health Survey (DHS) in 2008 recorded a national obesity prevalence of 9 percent among 15-49 year old women (Aryeetey and Ansong, 2011).

In Ghana very little is known about childhood and adolescent obesity. However, data gathered by the Ghana Demographic and Health Survey show that the prevalence of obesity within this population increased from 0.5 percent in 1988 to 1.9 percent in 1993 (de-Graft Aikins, 2007; GSS et al., 2004). Between 2003 and 2008 the prevalence of obesity among the youth aged 15–19 and 20–24 increased from 7.2 percent to 9.0 percent and 15.1 percent to 16.6 percent respectively (Dake et al., 2010). There are health implications of childhood obesity for the prevalence of certain diseases particularly chronic NCDs (Peltzer and Pengpid 2011). Some studies have indicated that childhood obesity is associated with a higher chance of obesity, premature death and disability in adulthood (Biritwum et al., 2005; Caprio et al., 2008; Berge et al., 2010).

Gender differences in prevalence have been reported, with obesity rates being higher among women than among men in Ghana. This is in contrast with data from high-income countries where obesity prevalence among men and women is comparable (Biritwum et al., 2005). Occupational differences have also been associated with obesity risk. A study by Aryeetey and Ansong

(2011) showed that among 141 workers of the College of Health Sciences of the University of Ghana, about 13 percent were found to be obese. It was also found that among urban civil servants in Ghana, the risk of abdominal obesity increased significantly with increasing levels of employment and wealth status (Amoah, 2003). In the same study, overweight and obesity were also found to be high among people who were in the service industry while among people who engaged in manual labour such as unskilled workers, farmers and fishermen, it was low.

There are ethnic differences in obesity prevalence. For instance, a study by Amoah (2003) reported high obesity rates among the Akan and Ga. Dake et al., (2010) showed that there has been a significant increase in obesity cases among Ga, Akan and Ewe people who mainly reside in urban southern Ghana. This supports the suggestion that obesity cases are higher among certain ethnic groups in Ghana. The underlying reasons for these differences – for example the genetic aspects - have not been fully explored (Biritwum et al., 2005).

Smoking

Although research on smoking in Ghana is limited, the available evidence suggests that the prevalence of tobacco use or smoking in Ghana is relatively low compared to other countries in sub-Saharan Africa. For example, the prevalence of smoking in South Africa and Tanzania was 34.4 percent and 27 percent respectively (Townsend et al., 2006; Jagoe et al., 2002) compared to the smoking prevalence of 9 percent in Ghana (Owusu-Dabo et al., 2009). This suggests that the expected epidemic rise in smoking prevalence has not occurred (Owusu-Dabo et al., 2009).

Regardless of the relatively low reported smoking prevalence in Ghana, smoking does occur especially among the adult population. In Ghana, studies have shown that modifiable risk factors such as tobacco use or smoking is usually common in urban areas compared with semi-urban or rural settings. The higher prevalence of smoking in urban areas is likely to contribute a significant risk to NCDs and is therefore likely to also increase the prevalence in such settings (See Addo et al., Chapter 1, de-Graft Aikins et al., Chapter 2).

Addo et al., (2006) found a hypertension prevalence of 25.4 percent among 362 respondents in four rural communities in the Ga District of the Greater Accra Region. In the study, the odds of developing hypertension among smokers were almost three times that of nonsmokers' odds.

Another study by Agyemang (2005) in Accra, Kumasi and four villages in the Ashanti Region showed an overall prevalence of hypertension to be 29.4 percent. In that study, smoking measured by current smoking status was independently associated with systolic and diastolic blood pressure, but only in men. In the same study, living in urban settings was also independently associated with high blood pressure. It has been suggested that smoking or the use of tobacco explains the urban and rural differences in NCD risk ,particularly hypertension (Kinra et al., 2010).

Tagoe and Dake (2011) conducted a secondary analysis of data from the World Heath Survey (WHS) in 2003 and the Ghana Demographic and Health Survey (DHS) of 2008. The study revealed a decreasing trend in smoking among Ghanaians from 12.4 percent (men) and 1.3 percent (women) in 2003 to 9.0 percent (men) and 0.5 percent (women) in 2008. A separate but smaller study by Owusu-Dabo et al., (2009) in the Ashanti region of Ghana among 6,258 respondents revealed that the prevalence of self-reported current smoking was 3.8percent (males 8.9 percent, females 0.3 percent) and of ever smoking 9.7 percent (males 22.0 percent, females 1.2 percent) thus corroborating the decreasing trend observed from the DHS data. In the latter study, smoking was more common in older people, those of low educational level, the unemployed and the less affluent. The study also revealed that smokers were more likely to drink alcohol and to have friends who smoke. The incidence of smoking has been linked with the increased likelihood of developing NCDs such as cancers, diabetes and hypertension over a period of time.

The Ghana report of the Global School Health Survey (GSHS) in 2007, showed that across Ghana, 1.5 percent of the 7,137 students interviewed indicated that they smoked cigarettes on one or more days during the last 30 days preceding the survey. Of the survey population, 5.1 percent had used tobacco in different forms, such as snuff powder, chewing tobacco, paper rolled tobacco, cigars or pipe on one or more days during the last 30 days preceding the survey.

Alcohol consumption

Alcohol consumption typically refers to the intake of an alcoholic drink. Alcohol overconsumption is usually defined as consuming an average of more than two alcoholic drinks per day for men and an average of more than one alcoholic drink per day for women. One drink is considered to be 355 ml regular beer, 148 ml wine, or 44 ml distilled spirits (Dufour, 1999)

It has been estimated that the annual per capita consumption of alcohol in Ghana is approximately 1.54 litres of pure alcohol (Evans, 2008). Locally manufactured alcoholic drinks account for 88 percent of consumption, with the remaining 12 percent coming from imports (Sutton and Kpentey, 2012). The locally brewed alcoholic beverages like palm wine, pito (millet wine) and *akpeteshie* (local gin) are among the most common alcoholic drinks in Ghana.

The focus of most surveys in Ghana on alcohol consumption has been the frequency and quantity of alcohol rather than the type of alcoholic beverage consumed by the respondent.

Results from the study by Tagoe and Dake (2011) indicated that more men and women reported consuming alcohol in Ghana in 2008 (32.7 percent and 15.4 percent respectively) than in 2003 (30.4 percent and 13.5 percent respectively). This suggests that the level of alcohol consumption as (measured by current consumption) among Ghanaian adults is on the increase and this is likely to increase the prevalence or burden of NCDs in Ghana. In the second round of the RIPS Urban Health and Poverty Survey, data analyses showed that among adults, current drinkers of alcohol (as measured by the consumption pattern) had a higher risk of hypertension than non-drinkers of alcohol (Awuah et al., submitted).

In the Ghana report of the GSHS, the prevalence of current alcohol use among students was found to be 15.3 percent. The report further indicated that of the students who had at least one drink containing alcohol during the 30 days preceding the survey, 14.6% reported usually drinking two or more drinks per day on the days they drank alcohol. In that survey, 6.9 percent of students reported being drunk on one or more occasions over the previous 30 days. Two percent of students reported that most or all of their friends drank alcohol and 4.3 percent reported that their parents drank alcohol. Kabiru et al., (2010) also conducted a secondary analysis of a nationally representative data collected from 4,430 adolescents aged 12-19 and they found that 9 percent of adolescents in Ghana reported that they had been drunk on at least one occasion in the 12 months preceding the survey.

It has been established that alcohol dependence is a major risk factor for chronic liver diseases including cirrhosis and may predispose one to liver cancer (Thun et al., 1997). Furthermore, alcohol dependence has been associated with thiamine deficiency and Korsakoff's syndrome, a form of mental disorder. A combination of alcohol use and other risk factors may also increase risk of cardiovascular disease. There is therefore a need for educational interventions with a focus on behavioural and lifestyle modification to help address alcohol-related issues. Relevant research is currently lacking in Ghana.

Physical inactivity

Physical activity is any movement in the body which is produced by skeletal muscles usually requiring the expenditure of energy (WHO, 2004). Physical inactivity or sedentary habits are associated with an increased risk of numerous chronic diseases and decreased longevity (Pate et al., 1995). Physical inactivity has been identified as the one of the leading risk factors for global mortality (WHO, 2004). Studies have shown that regular physical activity of moderate-to-vigorous intensity such as brisk walking and cycling, have significant benefits for health and can reduce the risk of NCDs (Moore et al., 2012). Physical activity can be measured in three domains: activity at work, travel to and from places and recreational activities (WHO, 2009).

The level of physical activity, especially among urban dwellers in Ghana, is low mainly due to sedentary lifestyles, modernization and migration. In the WHS (2003) and GDHS (2008), more than half of women and men (58.2 percent and 53.0 percent respectively) in Ghana had little or no physical activity in the days preceding the survey (Tagoe and Dake, 2011). Analysis of data gathered on youth (aged 15-24) in the RIPS Urban Health and Poverty Survey, showed that more than half (58.2 percent) were physically inactive (as measured by recreational activities) in the seven days preceding the survey (Afrifa-Anane et al., submitted). In the survey, analysis of data on the adult population in their reproductive ages (15-49 for women and 15-59 for men), showed that 30 percent were physical inactive (less than three days of household level physical activity). In that same study, respondents who had less than three days of physical activity were found to have elevated blood pressure compared to those who had three or more days of physical activity. A regression analysis showed that this relationship was statistically significant (Awuah et al., submitted). This implies that some level of physical activity, which can be achieved by all groups of people, should be promoted in intervention programmes.

Conclusion

There is a rising prevalence of the modifiable risk factors for chronic NCDs in Ghana as evidenced by population and community-based studies. The current prevalence of chronic NCDs, particularly in urban areas, is already as high as those seen in developed countries. In the absence of effective prevention measures, the prevalence of the modifiable risk factors of NCDs especially in low- and middle-income countries like Ghana, is likely to increase even further (Chobanian et al., 2003).

Evidence from observational studies in Ghana suggests that obesity rates have increased over the years, with more women likely to be obese than men. However, it is worth noting that most of the studies on obesity have tended to focus more on women than men. Even though rates of obesity in Ghana are lower for men than women, obese men are more likely to develop NCDs over time because of other risk factors such as smoking and alcohol consumption which are associated more with men than with women (Verbrugge, 1985; Waldron, 1983). The evidence also suggests that the youth or adolescents in Ghana are adopting lifestyles that could potentially increase their risk of chronic NCDs especially in adulthood.

We recommend that future research, partiularly, on obesity and its associated chronic NCDs in Ghana, should also focus on men. Additionally, there is a lack of data and/or research on risk factors such as alcohol overconsumption, smoking and physical inactivity even though the scarce research/data on these risk factors indicate that they are areas of concern. The majority of modifiable risk factors relate to physical inactivity and other aspects of lifestyle that favour obesity and NCDs. For these to be effectively addressed, multidisciplinary interventions are required to stem the increasing rates of NCDs in urban settings. Additionally, alcohol consumption and smoking, especially among men, should be addressed. The increasing levels of obesity, particularly among women and people engaged in sedentary occupations and lifestyle require further research. The associations between ethnicity and risk suggest that the socio-cultural dimensions of NCD risk factors need to be better understood.

Despite the increasing prevalence of NCD risk factors and the implications for morbidity and mortality, they have received very little attention from policy makers and political leaders (see Bosu, Chapter 9). It would be important for stakeholders to recognize the implications of a growing NCD epidemic in Ghana and to adopt practical ways of dealing with the risk factors. Population and community-based interventions are urgently needed to prevent and control NCDs for the general population, as well for individuals living with NCDs.

Table 7.1: Studies on Prevalence of NCD risk factors

Author(s)	Year of field work	Study population	Sample size	Age range	Response rate %	Method	Prevalence of Hypertension	Prevalence of Diabetes	Prevalence of Other NCD	Prevalence of Obesity
Kunutsor and Powles	2007	Kassena-Nankana District	574	18-65	95.7%	Cross-sectional survey	19.3%	-	-	-
Tagoe and Dake	2003 and 2008	Ghana	2,797 (2003) and 7,809 (2008)	18-49	-	Cross-sectional survey	-	-	-	-
Global school-based student health survey	2007	Ghana	7,137	-	81%	Cross-sectional survey	-	-	-	-
Kabiru et al.	-	Ghana	4,430	12-19	-	Cross-sectional survey	-	-	-	-
Agyeman	2004	Ashanti Region	1,431		82%-95%	Cross-sectional survey	29.4%	-	-	-
Darko	2008/9	Accra	2,814	18+	-	Mixed	27%	-	-	-
Peltzer and Pengpid	2007	Ghana	5,613		83%	Cross-sectional survey	-	-	-	-
Agyemang et al.	2004	Ashanti Region	1,277	8-16	-	Cross-sectional survey	-	-	-	-
Cappuccio et al.	2001	Ashanti Region	1,013	-	40% - 88%	Cross-sectional survey	28.7%	-	-	-
Addo et al.	-	Rural Accra	362	18+	60%-80%	Cross-sectional survey	25.4%	-	-	-

Author(s)	Year of field work	Study popu-lation	Sample size	Age range	Response rate %	Method	Preva-lence of Hyperten-sion	Preva-lence of Diabe-tes	Preva-lence of Other NCD	Preva-lence of Obesity
Owusu-Dabo et al.	-	Ashanti Region	6,258	14-105	-	Cross-sectional survey	-	-	-	-
Awuah et al.	2011	Accra	714	18-59	-	Cross-sectional survey	28.3%	-	-	-
Duda et al.	2005	Accra	305	18+	-	Cross-sectional survey	-	-	-	34.8%
Abubakari et al.	2000-2004	Ghana	-	15+	-	-	-	-	-	10%
Benkeser et al.	2008-2009	Accra	2,813	18+	-	Cross-sectional survey	-	-	-	31.1%
Biritwum et al.	2003	Ghana	4,231	18+	-	Cross-sectional survey	-	-	-	5.5%
Agyemang et al.	2004	Ashanti Region and the Netherlands	-		82%-95%	Cross-sectional survey	-	-	-	-
Escalona et al.	2000-2002	Accra	598	15+	-	Cross-sectional survey	-	-	-	17.2%

References

Abanilla, P.K., Huang,, K.Y., Shinners, D., Levy, A., Ayernor, K., de-Graft Aikins, A. and Ogedegbe G. (2011). Cardiovascular disease prevention in Ghana: feasibility of a faith-based organizational approach. *Bull World Health Organ*. 89:648–656.

Abubakari, A.R., Lauder, W., Agyemang,C., Jones, M., Kirk, A., and Bhopal, R.S. (2008).Prevalence and time trends in obesity among adult West African populations: a meta-analysis. *Obesity Reviews*. 9: 297-311.

Addo, J., Smeeth. L. and Leon, D.A. (2009). Obesity in urban civil servants in Ghana: Association with pre-adult wealth and adult socio-economic status. *Public Health*. 123:365-370.

Addo, J., Amoah, A.G.B. and Koram, K.A. (2006).The changing patterns of hypertension in Ghana: a study of four rural communities in the Ga district. *Ethn Dis*, 16: 894-899.

Afrifa-Anane, E., Codjoe, S.N.A., Agyemang, C., Ogedegbe,G. and de-Graft Aikins. The association of physical activity, body mass index and the blood pressure levels among youth in Accra, Ghana. In Preparation.

Agyemang, C., Owusu-Dabo, E., de Jonge, A., Martins. D., Ogedegbe, G. and Stronks K. (2008). Overweight and obesity among Ghanaian residents in The Netherlands: how do they weigh against their urban and rural counterparts in Ghana? *Public Health Nutrition*.12(7): 909-916.

Agyemang, C. (2006). Rural and urban differences in blood pressure and hypertension in Ghana, West Africa. *Public Health*. 120: 525-533.

Agyemang, C., Redekop,W.K., Owusu-Dabo, E. and Bruijnzeels,M.A. (2005) Blood pressure patterns in rural, semi-urban and urban children in the Ashanti region on Ghana, West Africa. *BMC Public Health*.2005;5:(114).

Agyei-Mensah S. and de-Graft Aikins A. (2010). Epidemiological transition and the double burden of disease in Accra, Ghana. *Journal of Urban Health* . 87 (5): 879-897.

Albu, J.B., Murphy. L., Frager. D.H., Johnson, J.A., Pi-Sunyer, F.X. (1997).Visceral fat and race-dependent health risks in obese nondiabetic premenopausal women. *Diabetes*. 46:456-462.

Alwan A (2008). 2008–2013 action plan for the global strategy for the prevention and control of non-communicable diseases. Report World Health Organization.

Amoah, A.G.B. (2003). Hypertension in Ghana: a cross-sectional community prevalence study in Greater Accra. *Ethn Dis*. 13:310 –315.

Amoah A. (2003). Sociodemographic variations in obesity among Ghanaian adults. *Public Health Nutrition*. 6 (8): 751- 757.

Aryeetey R and Ansong J. (2011). Overweight and hypertension among college of health sciences employees in Ghana. *AJFAND*. 11(6): 5444-5456.

Awuah, R.B., Anarfi,J.K., Agyemang,C., Ogedegbe,G., de-Graft AikinsA. Prevalence, awareness,treatment and control of hypertension in urban poor communities in Accra, Ghana. Submitted.

Benkeser, R.M., Biritwum, R., Hil, A.G.(2012). Prevalence of Overweight and Obesity and Perception of Healthy and Desirable Body Size in Urban, Ghanaian Women. *Ghana Med J.* 46(2): 66–75.

Berge JM, Wall M, Loth K and Neumark-Sztainer D (2010). Parenting style as a predictor of adolescent weight and weight –related behaviors. *Journal of Adolescent Health* Vol. 46: 331-338.

Biritwum, R.B., Gyapong, J., Mensah, G.(2000). The epidemiology of obesity in Ghana. *Ghana Med J.* 5 39(3):82-85.

Burke, V., Beilin, L.J., Simmer, K., Oddy, W.H., Blake. K.V., Doherty. D., Kendall G.E., Newnham. .JP., Landau, L,I., Stanley. F.J. (2005). Predictors of body mass index and associations with cardiovascular risk factors in Australian children: a prospective cohort study. *Int J Obes.* 19: 15 – 23.

Caballero B. (2007).The global epidemic of obesity: an overview. *Epidemiology Reviews.* 29: 1-5.

Cappuccio, F., Micah, F., Emmett, L., Kerry, S., Antwi, S., Martin- Peprah, R., Phillips, R, et al. (2004). Prevalence, detection, management and control of hypertension in Ashanti, West Africa. *Hypertension.* 1071-1021.

Caprio, S., Daniels, S.R., Drewnowski, A., Kaufman,F.R., Palinkas, L.A., Rosenbloom A.L. and Schwimmer, J.B. (2008). Influence of race, ethnicity, and culture on childhood obesity: implications for prevention and treatment. *Diabetes Care.* 31(11) pp: 2211 – 2221.

Chobanian, A.V., Bakris, G.L., Black, H.R., Cushman W.C., Green L.A., Izzo J.L. Jr, et al. (2003). The Seventh Report of the Joint National Committee on Prevention, Detection, Evaluation, and Treatment of High Blood Pressure: the JNC 7 report. *JAMA.* 289:2560–2572.

Darko, R., Adanu, R.M, Duda,R.B., Douptcheva, N, Hill, A.G.(2012). The health of adult women in Accra, Ghana: self-reporting and objective assessments 2008-2009. *Ghana Med J.* 46:2.

Dake, F.AA., Tawiah, E.O., Badasu, D.M. (2010). Sociodemographic correlates of obesity among Ghanaian women. *Public Health Nutrition:* 14(7): 1285–1291.

de-Graft Aikins, A. (2003). Living with diabetes in rural and urban Ghana: a critical social psychological examination of illness action and scope for intervention. *J Health Psychol.* 8(5): 557-572.

de-Graft Aikins, A.(2004). Strengthening quality and continuity of diabetes care in rural Ghana: a critical social psychological approach. *J Health Psychol.* 9(2): 295-309.

de-Graft Aikins, A. (2007). Ghana's neglected chronic disease epidemic: a developmental challenge. *Ghana Med J.* 41(4): 154-159.

de-Graft Aikins, A., Addo, J., Ofei, F., Bosu, W.K., Agyemang, C.(2012). Ghana's burden of chronic non-communicable diseases: future directions in research, practice and policy. *Ghana Med J.* 46 (2) suppl.

de-Graft Aikins, A, Anum A, Agyemang C, Addo J. Ogedegbe O. (2012).Lay representations of chronic diseases in Ghana: Implications for primary prevention. *Ghana Med J.* ; 46 (2) Suppl

de-Graft Aikins, A, Awuah RB, Pera T, Mendez M, Tran N, Zawada N. Explanatory models of Type 2 diabetes among people with Type 2 diabetes in urban poor communities in Accra, Ghana. Submitted.

Dickerson, J., Smith, M,. Benden, M., Ory, M. (2011). The association of physical activity, sedentary behaviours, and body mass index classification in a cross-sectional analysis: are the effects homogenous? *BMC Public Health.* 11 (926).

Duda, R.B., Darko, R., Seffah. J., Adanu, R.M.K., Anarfi, J.K., Hill, A.G. (2007). Prevalence of Obesity in Women of Accra, Ghana. *Afr J Health Sci.* 14: 154-159

Duda, R.B., Jumah, N.A., Hill, A.G., Seffah. J., Biritwum. R.(2006).Interest in healthy living outweighs presumed cultural norms for obesity for Ghanaian women. *Health Qual life Outcomes.* 4: 44.

Dufour, M.C., (1999).What Is Moderate Drinking? Defining "Drinks" and Drinking Levels. *Alcohol Research & Health* . 23 (1):5-14

Dupres, J.P., Nadeau, A., Tremblay, A. (1989). Role of deep abdominal fat in the association between regional adipose tissue distribution and glucose tolerance in obese women. *Diabetes.* 38:304-309.

Evans, K. (2008). National Alcohol Policy, third draft (13 May). Report prepared for the government of Ghana.

Garrow, J.S. (1988).Obesity and related diseases. London, Churchill Livingstone: 1-16.

Ghana Statistical Service (GSS), Noguchi Memorial Institute for Medical Research (NMIMR), and ORC Macro, 2004. Ghana Demographic and Health Survey 2003.Calverton, Maryland: GSS, NMIMR, and ORC Macro.

Holdsworth M, Gartner A, Landais E, Maire B, Delpeuch F (2004). Perceptions of health and desirable body size in urban Senegalese women. *Int J Obes Relat Metab Disord.* 28:1561-1568.

Isidoro, B., Lope, V., Pedraz-Pingarron, C., Collado-Garcia, F., Santamarina, C., Moreo, P. et al. (2001). Validation of obesity based on self-reported data in Spanish women participants in breast cancer screening programmes. *BMC Public Health.* 11:960

Jagoe K, Edwards R, Mugusi F, Whiting D, Unwin N. (2002). Tobacco smoking in Tanzania, East Africa: Population based smoking prevalence using expired alveolar carbon monoxide as a validation tool. Tob Control. 11(3): 210–214.

Kunustor, S. and Powels, J. (2009).Descriptive epidemiology of blood pressure in a rural adult population in northern Ghana. *Rural and Remote Health.* 9 (1025): 2-4.

Kabiru, C.W., Beguy, D., Crichton, J., Ezeh, A.C. (2010). Self-reported drunkenness among adolescents in four sub-Saharan African countries: Associations with adverse childhood experiences. *Child Adolesc Psychiatry Ment Health.* 4:17.

Kinra, S., Bowen, L.J., Lyngdoh. T., Prabhakaran, D., adjunct professor, Reddy, K.S., Ramakrishnan, L. et al. (2010). Sociodemographic patterning of non-communicable disease risk factors in rural India: a cross sectional study.*BMJ.* 341

Lemieux, S., Prud'homme, D., Bouchard, C., Tremblay, A., Després, J.P. (1993). Sex differences in the relation of visceral adipose tissue accumulation to total body fatness. *Am J Clin Nutr.* 58:463-467.

Moore, S.C., Patel, A.V., Matthews, C.E., Berrington de Gonzalez, A., Park, Y. et al. (2012.). Leisure Time Physical Activity of Moderate to Vigorous Intensity and Mortality: A Large Pooled Cohort Analysis. *PLoS Med.* 9(11)

Owusu-Dabo, E., Lewis, S., McNeill, A., Gilmore, A., Britton, J. (2009). Smoking uptake and prevalence in Ghana. *Tobacco Control.* 18:365–370.

Owusu-Dabo, E., Lewis, S., McNeill, A., Anderson, S., Gilmore. A., Britton, J. (2009). Smoking in Ghana: a review of tobacco industry activity. *Tobacco Control.* 18:206–211.

Popkin, B.M., Gordon-Larsen, P. (2004). The nutrition transition: worldwide obesity dynamics and their determinants. *Int J Obes Relat Metab Disord.* 28:S2-9.

Pate, R.R., Pratt, M., Blair, S.N. et al. *(1995). Physical activity and public health: a recommendation from the Centers for Disease Control and Prevention and the American College of Sports Medicine. JAMA.* 273:402–7.

Peltzer, K. and Pengpid, S. (2011). Overweight and obesity and associated factors among school- aged adolescents in Ghana and Uganda. *Int J Environ Res Public Health.* 8: 3859- 3870.

Sutton, .J and Kpentey, B. (2012). An Enterprise map of Ghana. International Growth Centre. London Publishing Partnership. pp. 77-85

Tagoe, H.A. and Dake, F.A.A. (2011). Healthy lifestyle behaviour among Ghanaian adults in the phase of a health policy change. *Globalization and Health.* 7(1): 7.

Thun, M.J., Peto, R., Lopez, A.D. et al. (1997). Alcohol consumption and mortality among middle-aged and elderly U.S. adults. *N Engl J Med .* 337:1705-14.

Townsend, L., Flisher, A.J., Gilreath, T., King, G. (2006). A systematic review of tobacco use among sub-Saharan Africa youth. *J Subst Use.* 11(4):245-269.

Verbrugge LM.(1985). Gender and health: an update on hypotheses and evidence. *J Health Soc Behav.*. 26: 156-182

Waldron I. (1983). Sex differencs in illness, incidence,prognosis and mortality: issues and evidence. *Soc Sci Med.* 17:1107-1123

World Health Organization (!995). Physical Status: the use and interpretation of anthropometry. Report of a WHO Expert Committee. Geneva, World Health Organization, (WHO Technical Report Series, No. 854).

World Health Organization. (2004). Appropriate body mass index for Asian populations and its implications for policy and intervention strategies. *Public Health The Lancet.* 363.

World Health Organization. (2011). Global status report on noncommunicable diseases 2010. WHO. 2011.

World Health Organization. (2009). Global Physical Activity Surveillance. Available from: http://www.who.int/chp/steps/GPAQ/en/index.html. WHO, 2009 [cited on June 13, 2013]

World Health Organization. (2005). Preventing Chronic Disease. A vital investment. Geneva: WHO.

World Health Organization. (2004) Global Strategy on Diet, Physical Activity and Health. WHO.

Chapter 8

The socio-cultural and socio-economic context of Africa's chronic disease burden[1]

Ama de-Graft Aikins

Introduction

Chronic disease risk and experiences are shaped by socio-cultural and socio-economic factors. There is a consensus that these dimensions require more research and nuanced understanding to facilitate the development of successful primary, secondary and tertiary interventions (Belue et al., 2010; de-Graft Aikins et al., 2010; Whyte, 2012). In this chapter I review the evidence on the socio-cultural and socio-economic dimensions on NCD risk and experiences in sub-Saharan Africa. The chapter is presented in four parts. In Part one I outline the evidence on the prevalence of the major non-modifiable risk factors: poor diets, physical inactivity, obesity, and other lifestyle practices such as smoking and alcohol overconsumption. In Part two I review the socio-cultural dimensions of these risk factors, focusing on socio-cultural meanings and norms relating to risk factors including diet, food practices and exercise. In Part three I present evidence on the social knowledge of the common NCDs and discuss the context shaping everyday illness experiences and health-seeking behaviour through the concepts of social logic and medical logic. The final section focuses on the socio-economic context of NCDs and considers the implications of urban poverty on illness experience and prognosis. I conclude by considering the implications of the existing evidence on the socio-cultural and socio-economic dimensions of NCDs on future research and interventions.

---

1   This is a modified version of what appeared as Chapter 2 in *Africa's Neglected Epidemic: Multidisciplinary research, intervention and policy for chronic diseases*, a peer-reviewed report of a conference convened by the British Academy, Royal Society and Ghana Academy of Arts and Sciences. The report was prepared by Ama de-Graft Aikins and can be accessed at www.britac.ac.uk. The modifications include an introduction, conclusions and the addition of newer relevant references.

Prevalence of modifiable chronic disease risk factors

Chronic diseases have non-modifiable and modifiable risks. The non-modifiable risks or 'inherent factors' are age and genetics. The modifiable risks include poor diets (lacking fruit and vegetables and high in saturated fats and salt), physical inactivity, obesity, high blood pressure and lifestyle practices such as cigarette smoking and high alcohol consumption. In many African countries the prevalence rates of these modifiable risk factors are high. A series of epidemiological survey has been conducted in African countries to examine the prevalence of risk factors of the major chronic diseases. Surveys include STEP Wise Surveys for NCD risk factor surveillance, Global Youth Tobacco Surveys, Global School Health Surveys, World Health Surveys and the Study of Global Ageing and Adult Health (SAGE) (see also Awuah and Afrifa-Anane, Chapter 7). These surveys show that physical activity is high in rural populations and low in urbanised populations in countries like Cameroon, Gambia, Ghana, Senegal and South Africa (Amoah, 2003; Steyn and Damasceno, 2006). Poor diets, low in fruits and vegetables and high in saturated fats, are more prevalent in urban settings (Steyn and Damasceno, 2006). Salt intake - a risk factor for hypertension - is high in both rural and urban populations in many countries (Cappuccio et al., 2000, 2006). Obesity rates are high and there are clear gender and urban rural differences in this area. Abubakari and colleagues (2008) conducted a meta-analysis of obesity among West African populations, and found obesity prevalence of 10.0 percent; women were more likely to be obese than men and urban populations had higher obesity rates than rural. Available data from Demographic and Health Surveys conducted in selected African countries show an accelerated increase in obesity prevalence among women over the last twenty years. In Ghana for example, obesity rates among women have tripled over 15 years: from 10 percent in 1993 to 30.5 percent in 2008 (GSS et al., 2004, 2009; see also Awuah and Afrifa-Anane, Chapter 7).

Smoking and alcohol intake rates vary across countries and are higher among male populations. Cigarette smoking is highest in South Africa and northern Africa; South Africa and northern African countries also record the highest rates of tobacco-related cancers (Parkin and Sasco, 1993). Countries like Ghana record low smoking rates, although there is an emerging trend of high smoking rates among the rural poor (Owusu-Dabo et al., 2009).

Adult per capita alcohol consumption is measured by dividing the sum of alcohol production and imports by alcohol exports by adult population aged

55 years and older (Baingana et al., 2006). Using this definition, alcohol consumption is reported to have increased in many African countries. Of the 13 countries with the highest recorded increase in global alcohol consumption between 1970 and 1996, five were African: Lesotho ranked 1st (with 1,817 percent increase), Nigeria ranked 5th (196 percent increase), Rwanda 10th, (129 percent increase) Burkina Faso, 12th (116 percent increase) and Sudan, 13th (108 percent increase). It is important to note that many African countries produce and consume home brews and spirits which are not taxable. This masks the true rate of alcohol consumption. However, similar profiles are found across countries: men drink more than women, the educated drink more than the uneducated, and there is a pattern of men drinking more frequently and binge drinking. In Namibia, Zimbabwe and Lesotho, there is increasing alcohol consumption among young people, below the age of 14 and as young as 5.

The socio-cultural context of modifiable chronic disease risks

There is increasing recognition that the socio-cultural context is an important mediating factor for chronic disease risks (Belue et al., 2009). Diet and food practices are major risk factors for the broad range of chronic diseases. Some traditional diets and traditional cooking and food preservation methods (e.g curing fish and meat with salt) contribute to the risk burden. However, the increased consumption of poor diets high in fat and processed nutrients in countries like Cameroon, Gambia, Ghana, Kenya, Senegal and Tanzania is more strongly associated with globalization, urbanization and Westernisation. In West Africa, food consumption patterns have changed from traditional diets high in locally produced coarse grains such as millet and sorghum to modern diets high in imported wheat and rice (Teklu, 1996). This change has been attributed to the aggressive marketing of processed foods by multinational food companies in the region. The interplay between structural and cultural factors must be understood in order to address the role of food practices in chronic disease risk.

Obesity has been highlighted as a cultural issue. High obesity rates among African women have been attributed to the associations many African societies make between fat, beauty, wealth and health (Prentice, 2006; Steyn and Damasceno, 2006). These associations have been reinforced by HIV/AIDS. Thinness is often associated with poverty and illness - and increasingly rapid and sustained weight loss is linked with HIV and AIDS in many countries.

Thus being plump or overweight is seen as a sign of being AIDS-free. Prentice (2006) argues that while Western countries stigmatise fat, this "psychological break" is missing in African countries. However, the evidence is mixed. While a study in Senegal showed that women preferred overweight BMI to normal BMI (Holdsworth et al., 2004), and a South African study suggested that black women did not perceive being overweight or obese as a health risk (Ndovlo et al., 1999), a study in Ghana suggests that "interest in healthy living outweighs presumed cultural norms for obesity"(Duda et al., 2006). Research in Ghana links female obesity to multiple child births and the obesogenic period of breastfeeding, when women face – and attempt to resist– cultural pressure to eat fatty foods and avoid strenuous activity, including exercise (de-Graft Aikins, 2011).

Concepts of exercise differ across cultures and societies. In Africa, daily physical activity is often linked to type of occupation. Rural farmers engage in strenuous physical activity as part of their work. Similarly in urban areas, there is high daily physical activity within the informal sector (e.g mechanics, street hawkers, domestic servants).Thus the available data on physical exercise makes rural-urban distinctions as well as distinctions between high physical activity among informal sector workers and low physical activity among salaried, sedentary workers in urban areas (Steyn and Damasceno, 2006).

The association between sports (such as football) or physical education in schools and high physical activity has not been explored in the literature on chronic disease risk factors. Research in this area is difficult due to the challenge of developing reliable and valid epidemiological methods that match self reports of physical activity to objective measures across different countries (Sobngwi et al., 2001).

Smoking and alcohol overconsumption have been identified as predominantly male problems and problems rooted in poverty. Culturally, many African societies frown on women smoking and drinking (Belue et al., 2009): thus female smoking and drinking may occur in secret. Poverty and poverty-related stresses (depression, anxiety, etc.) have physical and psychological health implications including the adoption of addictive behaviour like smoking, alcohol consumption and sexual promiscuity. Research on masculinity in South Africa shows that these addictive behaviour patterns confer a strong sense of masculinity, power and agency for men (Campbell, 2003).

Socio-cultural knowledge of chronic diseases

Research on hypertension, diabetes, stroke and cancers in Ghana, Cameroon and Tanzania highlight poor awareness and knowledge of the medical profile of these conditions (Awah et al., 2008; Clegg-Lamptey and Hodasi, 2007; de-Graft Aikins, 2005; Sitas et al., 2006). Late reporting of conditions like diabetes and cancers is common, although this might be a product of lay misdiagnosis as well as a lack of access to quality medical services. Late reporting compounds the rising prevalence of risk factors and of disease complications. For instance, 21 percent to 25 percent of type 2 diabetes patients have retinopathy at point of diagnosis.

Men and women with cancers report late for medical care, often at stages 3 and 4; their survival rate is poor (Clegg-Lamptey and Hodasi, 2007; Sitas et al., 2006). Cultural beliefs of the causes and consequences of chronic diseases have been implicated in poor illness practices. Anthropological research suggests that African societies subscribe to a tripartite model of disease. Illnesses can be naturally caused, socially caused, and/or spiritually and supernaturally caused (Senah, 2009; Mbiti 1964; Feierman and Janzen, 1991). Rare or unnatural events such as the death of a child or young adult, or chronic illnesses or illnesses which cause sudden death in otherwise healthy adults are often attributed to social or supernatural forces.

Studies on diabetes in Cameroon and Ghana show that lay communities and people with diabetes attribute diabetes to social and spiritual/supernatural causes, such as witchcraft (Awah et al., 2008; de-Graft Aikins, 2005). This leads some people with diabetes to healer-shop within ethnomedical and faith-healing systems. Spiritual causal theories are also implicated in the stigmatisation of people with diabetes and other serious chronic conditions, such as epilepsy (de-Graft Aikins, 2006; Allotey and Reidpath, 2007). However, cultural representations of health and disease are complex and research suggests that there are important dimensions of socio-cultural knowledge of chronic illness that can inform the development of effective primary and secondary interventions. First, research suggests that spiritual causal theories of chronic diseases are not universally dominant, nor do they lead to traditional medical practices in a linear way.

Research on social representations of diabetes in Ghana indicates that while people with diabetes may subscribe to spiritual causal theories, these theories co-exist with biomedical and psychological theories. This multi-level attribution process shapes complex illness practices within and across biomedical, ethnomedical and faith healing systems (de-Graft Aikins, 2005). Secondly, there is evidence that lay individuals possess some practical knowledge of major chronic diseases such as hypertension, diabetes and stroke (Awah et al., 2008; de-Graft Aikins et al., 2012; Kagee et al., 2007). This knowledge is drawn from a variety of medical and non-medical sources, including the mass media and churches. Ghanaian youth with Type 1 diabetes and their families, for example, identify the internet as an important source of information for disease management (Kratzer, 2012).

Finally, there are important cultural and ethnic variations in concepts of illness chronicity and incurability which may influence illness action strategies. In Ghana, some ethnic groups such as the Akan accommodate chronicity and have a term '*koa nkoro*' (literal translation 'difficult to fight') for this; other ethnic groups like the Ga do not (Atobrah, 2012; de-Graft Aikins et al., 2010). The term 'social logic' was coined by health psychologists to describe the way chronically ill individuals make sense of their illness and management routines by drawing on a broad repertoire of knowledge systems and material resources, including subjective and inter-subjective experiences, socio-cultural traditions and knowledge, social support and financial resources (de-Graft Aikins and Arhinful, 2009; Nettleton, 1995). Social logic enables the lay person to deal with the medical, psychological, spiritual, social and financial aspects of their condition. In contrast, health experts draw on 'medical logic' which is informed by a disease-centred approach to illness and focuses on a restricted repertoire of practical routines aimed at addressing the physiological dimension of the illness. Health promotion experts emphasise the importance of placing the complex and dynamic nature of social logic at the forefront of primary and secondary interventions.

Socio-economic context of chronic diseases: the role of poverty

The 'protracted polarised' process of epidemiological transition is evident in African countries with available data (Agyei-Mensah and de-Graft Aikins, 2010; Kahn et al., 2007; see Introduction to this volume). While chronic disease prevalence is higher among the urban wealthy in these countries, poor communities experience a 'double jeopardy' of chronic and infectious diseases. First, environmental pollution and degradation associated with poor rural and urban conditions of living are directly linked to diseases such as chronic respiratory disease (air pollution) and cancers (e-waste). Poverty and poor living conditions e.g. overcrowding, poor access to quality water - are also linked indirectly to chronic diseases, as the increased risk of infections and infectious diseases increases the risk of comorbid relationships between infectious and chronic diseases (e.g tuberculosis and diabetes, malaria and Burkitt Lymphoma). Secondly, poor communities experience high levels of undernutrition and malnutrition. Some studies show a relationship between maternal under-nutrition, low birth weight and later obesity and chronic disease risk for major conditions like atypical diabetes, cancers (stomach and oesophageal) and CVDs (rheumatic heart disease and dilated cardiomyopathy cardiovascular diseases) (Amuna, 2009).

Poor childhood nutrition, such as excessive consumption of sugar, heightens the risk of Type 1 and Type 2 diabetes. Thirdly, economic and psychosocial stresses associated with conditions of poverty are implicated in modifiable chronic disease risk factors such as smoking, excessive alcohol intake and unsafe sex. Finally, poor communities have poor access to healthcare: this has been categorised in terms of geographical (especially for poor rural communities), financial (travel costs and the high costs of medical consultation, drugs and new diets) and cultural (class and language barriers to effective health worker-client communication and relationships).

From the opposite end, the high cost of treating and managing chronic disease has a significant financial impact on individuals, families and households. WHO (2005) observes that 'chronic diseases can cause poverty in individuals and families, and draw them into a downward spiral of worsening disease and poverty' (p. 61). In Tanzania, in the 1990s, the cost of insulin (then $156 for a one-month supply) was beyond the means of the majority of Tanzanians (Chale et al., 1992) and the cost of diabetes care within the private health sector was 25 percent of the minimum wage (Neuhann et al., 2001). 'Catastrophic expenditures' for health care or 'impoverishing medical expenditures' constitute medical expenses that "endanger a household's ability to maintain its customary standard of living"(Suhrcke et al., 2006). A recent study in Burkina Faso demonstrated that the probability of catastrophic consequences increased by 3.3 to 7.8 times when a household member had a chronic illness (Tin Su et al., 2006).

In 2005, 388.03 million Africans - just over half of the continent's population - lived below the absolute poverty line of US$1.25 a day. In 2010, a little under half the continent's population – 48.5 percent - lived on US$1.25

a day. The majority of Africa's extreme poor lives in urban slum communities. Emerging research in urban slums shows high rates of chronic diseases and their complications (Kyobutungi et al., 2008). The relationship between rapid urbanization, extreme poverty and national chronic disease burdens should be a major issue for health policymakers and governments.

Conclusions

Chronic conditions are often described as diseases of lifestyle and, by extension, of wealth. Therefore, it is commonly assumed that chronic diseases are problems of wealthy nations and/or of wealthy communities in poor nations. This assumption is misleading. Wealth and poverty status may determine individual health. Similarly, individual lifestyle choices may predispose one to health or ill health. However, the roots of the global NCD burden move beyond individuals and their socio-economic status. Broader social, cultural and structural factors play important roles. As Hepworth (2004, pp.46-47) notes of the need for multi-level interventions for the global NCD burden: "health improvement requires strategies that encompass individual health knowledge, social relations (including medical relationships and communication), structural interventions such as legislation to ban smoking in public places and environmental factors such as pollution. This review has shown, for example, how poor communities face a double burden of infectious and chronic diseases due to a mix of socio-economic, lifestyle and environmental factors and how their poverty status raises their risk of avoidable chronic disease complications and deaths.

Similarly, experiences of NCDs move beyond the individual. Living with a chronic NCD in an African country involves living with and negotiating complex everyday challenges. The challenges are material and symbolic: they occur at the levels of the self, the significant other, medical systems, society, and the spiritual and supernatural realms. The challenges have implications for self-care, healthcare and long-term health and life outcomes. For example, although there is formal recognition of NCDs as a public health problem, there have been minimal policy investments in strengthening health systems to provide accessible, affordable and high-quality care. Therefore, most individuals struggle to access quality biomedical care. Biomedical deficiencies co-exist with a flourishing complementary health sector of competitive traditional medicine and faith-healing systems that offer unregulated and often harmful chronic disease care (de-Graft Aikins, 2005; Awah et al., 2008; Kolling et al., 2010).

These pluralistic medical systems enable and intensify healer-shopping. In terms of everyday experiences, individuals who live with conditions which share AIDS-like symptoms, like cancers and uncontrolled diabetes, are stigmatized. Supernatural causal theories of common NCDs may raise the risk of witchcraft accusations within families and communities. These material and symbolic challenges have implications for NCD risk, self-care, healthcare and long-term health and life outcomes. Therefore, interventions that seek to address NCD risk, morbidity and mortality in sub-Saharan Africa must incorporate the psychological, social, cultural and structural dimensions of the problem.

References

Abubakari, A., Lauder W, Agyemang C, Jones M, Kirk A, Bhopal RS: (2008). Prevalence and time trends in obesity among adult West African populations: a meta-analysis. *Obesity Review,* 9:297-311.

Agyei-Mensah, S. and de-Graft Aikins, A. (2010). Epidemiological transition and the double burden of disease in Accra, Ghana. *Journal of Urban Health. 87 (5), 879-897.*

Allotey, P. and Reidpath, D. (2007). Epilepsy, Culture, Identity and Wellbeing A Study of the Social, Cultural and Environmental Context of Epilepsy in Cameroon. *Journal of Health Psychology,* 12(3) 431–443.

Amoah, A.G.B. (2003). Sociodemographic variations in obesity among Ghanaian adults.*Public Health Nutrition,* 6(8): 751-775.

Amuna, P. (2009). Poverty and the biological basis of chronic disease in Africa. Paper presented at The British Academy, Royal Society and Ghana Academy of Arts and Sciences Conference, *Africa's Neglected Epidemic: Multidisciplinary Research,Intervention and Policy for Chronic Disease. Accra.*

Awah, P.K, Unwin, N. and Phillimore, P. (2008) Cure or control: complying with biomedical regime of diabetes in Cameroon. *BMC Health Services Research,* 8,43;

Baingana, F.K., Alem, A., and Jenkins, R. (2006). Mental health and the abuse of alcohol and controlled substances. In: Jamison, D.T., Feachem, R.G., Makgoba, M.W., Bos, E.R., Baingana, F.K., Hofman, K.J. and Rogo, K.O. (Eds). *Disease and Mortality in Sub- Saharan Africa.* (2nd Ed) Washington DC: The World Bank. (pp.329-350)

BeLue, R, Okoror, T.A., Iwelunmor. J., Taylor, K.D., Degboe, A.N., Agyemang, C, Ogedegbe, O. (2009). An overview of cardiovascular risk factor burden in sub-Saharan African countries: a socio-cultural perspective. *Globalization and Health,* 5:10;

Campbell, C (2003). *Letting them die: Why HIV/AIDS prevention programmes fail.* Oxford: James Curry.

Cappuccio, F.P., Plange-Rhule, Phillips, R.O, and J.B. Eastwood. (2000). Prevention of Hypertension and Stroke in Africa. *Lancet* 356:677-78.;

Cappuccio, F.P., Kerry, S.M., Micah F.B., Plange-Rhule, J., Eastwood J.B. (2006). A community programme to reduce salt intake and blood pressure in Ghana. *BMC Public Health.*6:13.

Chale, S., Swai, A., Mujinja, P. and MacLarty, D. (1992). Must diabetes be a fatal disease in Africa? Study of cost of treatment, *British Medical Journal,* 304:1215-1218.

Clegg-Lamptey, J.N.A., and Hodasi, W.M. (2007). A study of breast cancer in Korle-Bu Teaching Hospital: assessing the impact of health education. *Ghana Medical Journal*, 41(2), 72-77;

de-Graft Aikins, A (2005). Healer-shopping in Africa: new evidence from a rural-urban qualitative study of Ghanaian diabetes experiences. *British Medical Journal*, 331, 737;

de-Graft Aikins, A. (2006). Reframing applied disease stigma research: a multilevel analysis of diabetes stigma in Ghana. *Journal of Community and Applied Social Psychology*, 16(6), 426-441.

de-Graft Aikins, A (2011) Culture, diet and the maternal body: Ghanaian women's perspectives on food, fat and childbearing. In Maya Unnithan-Kumar and Soraya Tremayne (Eds). *Fatness and the Maternal Body: Women's experiences of corporeality and the shaping of social policy*. Oxford: Berghahn Books

de-Graft Aikins and Arhinful, D.K. (2009). Chronic Disease Intervention in Africa: bridging the gaps between theory, practice and policy. Paper presented at The British Academy, Royal Society and Ghana Academy of Arts and Sciences Conference, *Africa's Neglected Epidemic: Multidisciplinary Research, Intervention and Policy for Chronic Disease. Accra.*

de-Graft Aikins, A, Boynton, P. and Atanga, L.L. (2010). Developing Effective Chronic Disease Prevention in Africa: practical and theoretical insights from Ghana and Cameroon. *Globalization and Health.* 6:6.

Duda, R.B., Jumah, N.A., Hill, A.G., Seffah, J., and Biritwum, R. (2006). Interest in healthy living outweighs presumed cultural norms for obesity for Ghanaian women. *Health and Quality of Life Outcomes* 2006, 4:44

Frenk et al. (1989). Health Transition in middle-income countries: new challenges for health care. *Health Policy and Planning* 4 (1): 29-39.

Ghana Statistical Service (GSS), Noguchi Memorial Institute for Medical Research (NMIMR), and ORC Macro (2004). *Ghana Demographic and Health Survey 2003.* Calverton, Maryland: GSS, NMIMR, and ORC Macro;

Ghana Statistical Service (GSS), Noguchi Memorial Institute for Medical Research (NMIMR), and ORC Macro (2009). *Ghana Demographic and Health Survey 2008.* Calverton, Maryland: GSS, NMIMR, and ORC Macro.

Holdsworth, M., Gartner, A., Landais. E., Maire, B., Delpeuch, F. (2004). Perceptions of healthy and desirable body size in urban Senegalese women. *International Journal of Obesity*, 28(12):1561-1568.

Kagee, A., Le Roux, M., and Dick, J. (2007) Treatment Adherence among Primary Care Patients in a Historically Disadvantaged Community in South Africa. A Qualitative Study. *Journal of Health Psychology*, 12 (3), 444-460.

Kahn, K., Garenne, M.L., Collinson, M.A., Tollman, S.M. (2007). Mortality trends in a new South Africa: Hard to make a fresh start. *Scandinavian Journal of Public Health*, 35 (S69), 26-34;

Kratzer, J. (2012). Structural Barriers to coping with Type 1 Diabetes Mellitus in Ghana: experiences of diabetic youth and their families. *Ghana Medical Journal*. 46(2), 39-45.

Kruger HS, Puoane T, Senekal M, van der Merwe MT. (2005) Obesity in South Africa: challenges for government and health professionals. *Public Health Nutrition*, 8:491– 500.

Kyobutungi, C., Ziraba, A.K., Ezeh, A., and Ye, Y. (2008). The burden of disease profiles of residents in Nairobi slums: Results from a demographic surveillance system. *Population Health Metrics*, Vol 6, 1

Levine, C.E., Ruel, M.T., Morris, S.S., Maxwell, D.G., Armar-Klemesu, M, and Ahiadeke, C. (1999). Working women in an urban setting: Traders, Vendors and Food security in Accra. *World Development*, 27 (11), 1977-1991.

Mensah GA (2008). Epidemiology of stroke and high blood pressure in Africa. *Heart* 2008, 94:697-705.

Murray, C.J.L. and Lopez, A.D. (1997). Mortality by cause for eight regions of the world: Global Burden of Disease Study." *Lancet*, 349:1269-76.

Ndovlo, P.P. and Roos, S.D. (1999). Perceptions of Black Women of Obesity as a Health Risk. *Curationis*, 22 (2): 47-55.

Neuhann HF, C Warter-Neuhann, I Lyaruu and L Msuya, 2001. 'Diabetes care in Kilimanjaro region: clinical presentation and problems of patients of the diabetes clinic at the regional referral hospital – an inventory before structured intervention', *Diabetic Medicine* 19: 509–513.

Nettleton, S (1995). *The Sociology of Health and Illness*. Oxford: Polity

Omran, A.R. (1971). The epidemiological transition theory: a theory of the epidemiology of population change. *Milbank Memorial Fund Quarterly*, 49: 6-47.

Owusu-Dabo E, Lewis S, McNeill A, Anderson S, Gilmore A, Britton J. (2009). Smoking in Ghana: a review of tobacco industry activity. *Tobacco Control*. 18:206–211.

Parkin, D.M. and Sasco, A.J. (1993). Lung cancer: worldwide variation in occurrence and proportion attributable to tobacco use. *Lung Cancer*, 9: 1-16.

Prentice, A.M. (2006). The emerging epidemic of obesity in developing countries. *International Journal of Epidemiology*. 35, 93-99.

Senah, K. (2009). Lay community uses of plural medical systems Paper presented by Prof Kodjo Senah at The British Academy, Royal Society and Ghana Academy of Arts and Sciences Conference, *Africa's Neglected Epidemic: Multidisciplinary Research, Intervention and Policy for Chronic Disease.*

Sitas, F., Parkin, M., Chirenje, Z., Stein, L., Mqoqi, N. and Wabinga, H. (2006). Cancers. In Jamison, D.T., Feachem, R.G., Makgoba, M.W., Bos, E.R., Baingana, F.K., Hofman, K.J. and Rogo, K.O. (Eds). *Disease and Mortality in Sub-Saharan Africa*. (2nd Ed) Washington DC: The World Bank. (pp. 289-304)

Smallman-Raynor, M and Phillips, D. (1999). Late stages of epidemiological transition: health status in the developed world. *Health and Place*, 5, 209-222. (p. 211)

Sobgnwi, E., Mbanya, J.C., Unwin, N.C., Terrence, J.A., and Alberti, K.G.M.M. (2001). Development and validation of a questionnaire for the assessment of physical activity in epidemiological studies in sub-Saharan Africa. *International Journal of Epidemiology*, 30:1361-68.

Steyn, K. and Damasceno, A. (2006). Lifestyle and Related risk factors for chronic disease. In Jamison, D.T., Feachem, R.G., Makgoba, M.W., Bos, E.R., Baingana, F.K., Hofman, K.J. and Rogo, K.O. (Eds). *Disease and Mortality in Sub-Saharan Africa*. (2nd Ed) Washington DC: The World Bank. (pp.247-265)

Suhrcke M, Nugent RA, Stuckler D, Rocco L: *Chronic Disease: An Economic Perspective* London: Oxford Health Alliance; 2006.

Teklu, T. (1996). Food demands studies in sub-Saharan Africa: A survey of empirical evidence. *Food policy*, 21: 479-96.

Tin Su T, B Kouyaté and S Flessa, (2006). 'Catastrophic household expenditures for health care in a low income society: a study from Nouna district, Burkina Faso', *Bulletin of the World Health Organization* 84: 21–27.

Treloar, C., Porteous, J., Hassan, F., Kasniyah, N., Lakshmanudu, M., Sama, M., Sja'bani , M. and Heller, R.F. (1999). The Cross Cultural Context of Obesity: An INCLEN Multicentre Collaborative Study. *Health and Place*, 5:279-86;

UNFPA (United Nations Population Fund) (2000). *State of World Population*. New York: United Nations

Whyte, S.R (2012). Chronicity and control: framing 'noncommunicable diseases' in Africa. *Anthropology and Medicine*, 19:1, 63-74

WHO (2004).World Health Report. WHO, Geneva, Switzerland

WHO/FAO (2003). *Diet, nutrition and the prevention of chronic diseases: report of a joint WHO/FAO expert consultation*. Geneva: WHO.

Chapter 9

A comprehensive review of the policy and programmatic response to rising chronic non-communicable disease in Ghana[1]

William K. Bosu

Introduction

Although chronic non-communicable diseases (NCDs) have contributed significantly to Ghana's disease burden for more than fifty years, it is only in recent years that they have begun to capture national attention (Colbourne et al., 1950; Hill et al., 2007; Nyame et al., 1994; Pobee, 1993). In a survey in 1950 among 255 persons aged 0-75 years (95percent of them less than 50 years) in Kwansakrom, a village 60 miles from Accra, 14 (5.5 percent) were found to have cardiovascular disease with an organic cardiac murmur or a diastolic blood pressure of more than 100 mmHg (Colbourne et al., 1950). Over the period from 1960 to 1968, strokes accounted for 6-10 percent of deaths in adult patient and approximately 8 percent of medical admissions at the Korle-Bu Teaching Hospital (KBTH), Accra (Haddock, 1970). Between 1990 and 1993, the proportions increased to 17 percent and 11 percent respectively (Nyame et al., 1994).

The first major community-based systematic study of cardiovascular diseases was undertaken in Mamprobi, Accra in 1974-1976 by the University of Ghana Medical School with support from the World Health Organization (WHO). The study found that 25 percent of urban population aged 15-64 years had abnormal cardiovascular (CVD) findings (Ikeme et al, 1978). Thirteen percent of respondents had raised blood pressure ≥160/95 mmHg and 3.4 percent had rheumatic heart disease. In a five year follow up survey from 1975, CVDs accounted for 48 percent of the adult deaths in this community (Pobee, 1993, 2006). By 2003, an epidemic of chronic disease risk factor among women in

1   Previously published as Bosu. W.K (2012). A comprehensive review of the policy and programmatic response to chronic non-communicable disease in Ghana. *Ghana Medical Journal*, 46(2), 69-78.

Accra had emerged with 35 percent of them being obese, 40 percent hypertensive and 23 percent hypercholesterolaemic (Hill et al., 2007). In Accra, Kumasi and rural areas, the estimated adult prevalence of hypertension is 28-40 percent (Hill et al., 2007, Agyemang et al., 2006; Amoah, 2003; Cappuccio et al., 2004; Agyemang 2006). Nationally, hypertension has moved from being the ninth to tenth commonest cause of new outpatient morbidity in all ages in 1985-2001 to become the fifth since 2002. Stroke and hypertension have regularly been among the leading causes of deaths in hospitals in Ghana for more than 20 years. The estimated 6-7 percent adult prevalence of diabetes in Accra in 1998-2002 (Hill et al., 2007; Amoah et al., 2002) and 9.5 percent in Kumasi in 2005 (Owiredu et al., 2008), is markedly higher than previous estimates of 0.4 percent in 1956 (Dodu, 1958).

Consistent with the reported increases in chronic NCDs, obesity levels have also been increasing (Hill et al., 2007; GSS et al., 2009; Martorell et al., 2000) and fruit and vegetable consumption is among the lowest in Africa (Hall et al., 2009). In the face of the high and increasing burden of chronic NCDs in Ghana, this paper attempts to review the national policy response, examine achievements and current challenges and recommend options available to deal with the situation.

Methods

Unpublished reports, documents, files, letters were studied to identify programmatic issues at the Non-Communicable Disease Control Programme of the Ghana Health Service. Data extracted included the epidemiology of NCDs, the policy and programmatic responses and recommended strategies for prevention and management of NCDs. Data on the policy implications of chronic NCDs in Ghana were obtained from a search of the PubMed electronic database of published articles from 1970 to August 2009. In addition, the websites of various institutions such as the World Health Organisation (WHO) headquarters, WHO Regional Office for Africa, the Ministry of Health and the Ghana Health Service as well as media agencies were searched for relevant articles.

Results and discussion

Establishment of the Non-Communicable Diseases Control Programme

The establishment of the Burkitt's Lymphoma Centre at the Korle-Bu Teaching Hospital (KBTH) with support from the National Institute of Health, USA, was followed by attempts to establish a cancer registry in the early 1970s. However, these efforts were only partially successful due partly to leadership problems and the exodus of skilled practitioners. The efforts to address cancers and evidence of the growing importance of cardiovascular diseases in Ghana influenced the establishment of the Non-Communicable Diseases Control and Prevention (NCDCP) Programme in 1992 by the then Ministry of Health (MOH). The objectives of the programme were to reduce the incidence of NCDs, to reduce their morbidity, to prevent complications and disability from NCDs and to prolong the quality of life of individuals and the general population.

The diseases covered by the NCDCP include chronic NCDs with shared risk factors (cardiovascular disease, diabetes, cancers and chronic respiratory diseases), genetic disorders (sickle cell disease) and injuries. Tobacco control is not an integral part of the NCDCP, and is managed by the Health Research Directorate. There is also good collaboration with the Health Promotion Department and the Family Health Directorate with respect to health promotion programmes and the control and prevention of breast and female reproductive cancers.

The functions of the NCDCP include planning, advocacy, training, coordinating NCD-related activities, research, health communication, development of clinical practice guidelines, mobilizing resources for NCD prevention and control. There are only a few focal persons - for cancer, tobacco control and sickle-cell disease. The programme structure at the regional and district level is not as well defined. A pertinent problem is that the peripheral health priority actions are determined more by the availability of dedicated funds from 'vertical' programmes such as HIV, tuberculosis, immunization than by local disease profile.

Policy initiatives for NCDs: 1995-2008

Although NCDs were included in several health policy documents during the mid-1990s, practical attention to their control was hindered by low political will and limited funding. In 1994, MOH identified the development of more effective and efficient systems for the surveillance, prevention and control of communicable and non-communicable diseases of socio-economic importance as one of the main strategies to achieve its health service targets by the year 2000 (MOH, 1994). In 1995, MOH developed a major health strategy paper towards achieving the government's long-term developmental agenda, called Vision 2020, after a series of national consultations which started in September 1993. A package of priority health services including treatment of hypertension, diabetes, asthma, sickle cell disease, malnutrition and cancer was listed which should be accessible to the majority of Ghanaians (MOH, 1995). Despite the inclusion of NCDs in the priority list of diseases, the specific health strategies drawn up for Vision 2020 excluded control of NCDs (MOH, 1996). Moreover, except for the year 2000, the external annual independent reviews of the health sector performance of 1997-2003 hardly mentioned NCDs or proposed any recommendations for their prevention and control.

It was during the mid-term review of the Programme of Work (POW) 1997-2001 in 2000 that the burden of NCDs was discussed in the Health of the Nation Report (MOH, 2001). One background report catalogued interventions such as the development of a draft policy and programme document, the activities of the Ghana Diabetes Advisory Board inaugurated in 1997, the implementation of a comprehensive diabetes management programme in many hospitals in Ghana, screening programmes for breast cancer, cervical cancer and neonatal sickle cell disease in parts of Ghana, and the activities of NCD-specific peer non-governmental organizations (NGOs) (Health Interventions Group, 2001).

The establishment of the Ghana Health Service (GHS) and the Teaching Hospitals under Act 525 in 1996, at least in theory, provided service agencies as well as the regulatory bodies some administrative and financial autonomy to undertake their tasks. During the period of the POW 1997-2001, the major achievements in the prevention and control of NCDs included intense promotion of exclusive breastfeeding, passage of a legislative instrument on breastfeeding, introduction of a smoking ban in public health facilities, development of a strategy paper for NCDs, and the introduction of user fee exemption for persons older than 70. The University of Ghana Medical School developed national treatment guidelines and trained multidisciplinary teams in regions and districts to improve the care of diabetes from 1995-1998 with funding from Eli Lilly Company and MOH Ghana (Amoah et al., 2000). In 2001, a national conference was held to highlight the emerging epidemic of NCDs. A national NCD policy was drafted in 2002 (NCDCP, 2002). A national stakeholder's conference was also held to discuss the establishment of a national population-based cancer registry. Study visits were undertaken to Lyons (France) and Banjul to understudy cancer registration.

During the second GHS POW 2002-2006, NCDs became more nationally visible and were prioritized in the national health interventions due in part to the interests of the then Director-General of the GHS and the Minister of Health. Ironically, the POW 2002-2006, like its predecessor POW 1997-2001, was generally silent on NCDs. National and international events such as the World Diabetes Day, World No Tobacco Day, World Heart Day, were regularly celebrated during this period. Hepatitis B vaccine was introduced into the national immunization programme in 2002 to prevent virus-related liver cancer. The GHS lobbied Parliament to ratify the Framework Convention on Tobacco Control (FCTC) in 2004. Anti-tobacco activities were intensified, buoyed by the ban on public smoking in several European Union countries. A draft tobacco bill was presented to the Cabinet in 2005. Risk factors surveys were conducted by various groups in Accra and Kumasi to provide a better understanding of risk factors associated with hypertension (Cappuccio et al., 2004; Agyemang, 2006; Biritwum et al., 2005; Duda et al., 2007). The Demographic and Health Survey (DHS) in 2003 provided nationwide data on childhood and adult female obesity and tobacco use in males (GSS et al., 2004). The GDHS 2008 additionally provides information on alcohol, fruit and vegetable consumption (GSS et al., 2009).

Inspired by the government's vision to transform Ghana into a middle -income country by 2015, the then Minister of Health, Major Courage Quashigah (rtd) determined to create wealth through health. Following a visit to Dimona, Israel, in June 2005, and the observation of zero NCD cases or deaths among 4,000 African Hebrews in about 40 years, the Minister instituted a programme to re-orient Ghana's health policy to emphasise regenerative health promotion. In 2006, an agreement was signed requesting the African Hebrew Development Agency (ADHA) to work with MOH to design, pilot and scale up the implementation of a Regenerative Health and Nutrition Programme (RHNP)(AHDA, 2008). Contrary to its non-service delivery mandate, MOH established the RHNP in 2006 and has since been managing it. The strategic plan 2007-2011 of RHNP has four key areas: behaviour change communication, creating enabling environments, capacity building and training, and partnership and networking (MOH, 2008). The four priority RHNP interventions are: promoting healthy, largely plant-based diets; exercise; rest and environmental cleanliness. The Dimona model advocates regular colonic cleansing and drinking water about 30 minutes before meals. RHNP was initially piloted in 10 districts in seven regions and was favourably evaluated in 2007 (MOH, 2008a). More than 200 Ghanaians, including traditional rulers, actors, musicians and journalists have visited Dimona, to enable them learn more and promote regenerative health care.

In June 1995, the NCDCP organized a national seminar with the aim of creating awareness of NCDs and fostering better collaboration between clinicians and public health practitioners (MOH, 2005b). Ten years later in June 2005, the NCDCP organized a national stakeholders' conference covering the public health and social dimensions of cardiovascular diseases, diabetes, cancers, sickle cell disease, asthma and injuries (NCDCP, 2005). The objectives of the conference were to begin a process of developing a strategic framework for the control of NCDs, to design a plan to halt NCDs in Ghana and to review current strategies to prevent and control NCDs. There was consensus that an integrated approach and partnerships were essential strategies for the prevention and control of NCDs. Following the conference in 2006-2007, five technical working groups were constituted to develop draft strategic frameworks for the prevention and control of cardiovascular diseases, diabetes, cancers, asthma and sickle cell disease which are still being finalized.

By far the most relevant programme for NCDs in Ghana has been the current health sector POW 2007-2011, with the theme 'Creating Wealth through Health' (MOH, 2008b). Besides the prevailing paradigm shift from curative to preventive health policy and the establishment of the RHNP, the development of the third health sector POW was more consultative and engaged many GHS disease-control programmes. The four strategic objectives of the POW are to: promote an individual lifestyle and behavioural model for improving health and vitality by addressing risk factors and by strengthening multi-sectoral advocacy and actions; rapidly scale high impact interventions and services targeting the poor, disadvantaged and vulnerable groups; invest in strengthening health system capacity to sustain high coverage and expand access to quality of health services; and to promote governance, partnership and sustainable financing.

Consistent with the POW 2007-2011, the current health policy of Ghana clearly emphasises the promotion of healthy lifestyles and healthy environments and the provision of health, reproduction and nutrition services as two of seven priority areas of action (MOH, 2007). The policy further identifies six programme areas which will be emphasized and resourced in order to achieve the health sector objectives. Two of these programme areas are promoting good nutrition across the life span; and reducing NCD-related risk factors such as tobacco and alcohol use, lack of exercise, poor eating habits and unsafe driving.

Policy measures to be implemented towards achieving healthy lifestyles and healthy environments include developing standards and programmes for promoting healthy settings, as in healthy homes, schools, workplaces and communities (MOH, 2007). Healthy schools will be promoted through collaboration between the MOH, GES and private schools to facilitate the adoption of healthy lifestyles among students through the curriculum, physical education, environmental sanitation and the promotion of healthy eating. Ensuring food safety requires developing and enforcing standards for the production, storage, sale and handling of food and drink in markets, restaurants and through other vendors.

Strategies for prevention and control of NCDs – the international context

According to WHO, there have been more than 50 resolutions on chronic diseases prevention and health promotion since 1948 (http://www.who.int/nmh/about/en/). They cover issues such as tobacco control, diet, physical activity, nutrition, alcohol and sickle cell disease (Table 1). Notable among these are the Framework Convention on Tobacco Control (FCTC) of 2003 and the Global Strategy on Diet, Physical Activity and Health (DPAS) of 2004.

In May 2008, the Sixty-first World Health Assembly endorsed a six-year Global Action Plan 2008-2013 which provides Member States and the international community with a roadmap to establish and strengthen initiatives for the surveillance, prevention and management of NCDs (WHA61.14) (WHO, 2008).

Besides the numerous global resolutions, the WHO Regional Committee for Africa has, since 2000, also produced continent-specific guidelines for the prevention and control of NCDs (WHO-AFRO, 2000, 2005, 2007a, 2007b, 2007c, 2008a, 2008b). In 2006, the tenth ECOWAS Nutrition Forum acknowledged the 'double burden' of over- and under-nutrition in the sub-region, even in the same households (WAHO, 2006). The Ouagadougou Declaration of 2008 affirms that the overall strengthening of the health system provides the enabling environment for the prevention and control of NCDs (WHO, 2008). Despite the useful recommendations in these international resolutions,

Ghana, like other countries, does not appear to have an institutional framework to monitor the implementation of these international provisions.

National strategies for prevention and control of NCDs

Ghana has prepared a number of strategy papers. In 1993, the NCDCP described general strategies for the prevention and control of chronic NCDs as well as disease-specific strategies (Sackey, 1993). The paper proposed a two-phase implementation of the programme, from January 1994 to December 1998 and from January 1999 to December 2004, with specified targets for each phase. The roles and responsibilities of the national, regional, district, sub-district and community levels were specified. In 1998, another strategy paper was prepared with a view to documenting the burden of NCDs, identifying the risk factors and designining the most appropriate intervention packages for the Ghanaian situation (MOH, 1998). The aims were to: form a national NCDs Technical Advisory Board and expert technical sub-committees on the various NCDs; develop health educational materials and methodologies for NCDs; establish counselling, consultation units for NCDs in all Regional and District Hospitals; strengthen the capacity of health workers in NCD surveillance; strengthen the capacity of health teams in the knowledge, diagnosis, management and control of NCDs; develop and produce standardized management guidelines and protocols for NCDs; and conduct baseline research on the targeted NCDs.

In March 2002, a technical team prepared a draft national policy framework for NCDs with technical support from WHO but it was not formally adopted (MOH, 2002). The policy framework covered the justification for NCD prevention and control, strategic objectives, strategies, capacity building, drugs, health care costs and risk sharing, and monitoring and evaluation. In 2006-2007, strategic frameworks for the control of the major NCDs were developed. Finalization of these strategy documents is in progress. In 2008, the NCDCP prepared a position paper which assessed the current situation of NCDs in the country, the national response and proposed recommendations for improving the situation (Bosu, 2008). Implementation of the recommendations has been very slow, largely due to financial constraints and low resolve to do so. There is no national coordinating body to push for their implementation.

A combination of population-based (e.g. smoking ban in or around health facilities) and high risk-based strategies (low salt intake in hypertensives) are currently employed. Primary prevention strategies include advocacy for political support, legislation and health promotion emphasizing healthy lifestyles. Secondary prevention strategies include educational campaigns and screening for early detection (of overweight, raised blood pressure, raised cholesterol, and selected cancers) and development of clinical practice guidelines. Tertiary prevention aims to improve the quality of life of those with complications resulting from NCDs. This involves the use of prostheses, occupational therapy, speech therapy and palliative care. Cross-cutting strategies include training, human resource mobilization, research, supervision, partnerships and intersectoral collaboration. Priority interventions are preventive and are implemented through an integrated approach which targets major risk factors (WHO, 2008).

Status of recent policy implementation on NCDs and related challenges in Ghana

One of the main achievements has been the ratification of the Framework Convention on Tobacco Control (FCTC) and subsequent drafting of a national tobacco bill under the leadership of the Food and Drugs Board. Since 2005, the bill has been before Cabinet but there are now indications that the government would like to revise and pass it into law (GNA, 2009a). There are no clear laws on labelling of processed foods in Ghana and so the content of most processed foods are not labelled. Interestingly, products exported to Europe tend to be labelled. There are laws in place that are hardly enforced against advertisements claiming exaggerated health benefits (including aphrodisiac properties) of products such as alcoholic 'bitters' and herbal products. Neither is the law banning the sale of alcohol to under-aged persons.

Sensitization of the general public on healthy lifestyles has been improving due to health sector campaigns at all levels using the mass media. The NCD Control Programme has over the past five years organized sensitization workshops for regional health teams, media persons, and NGOs. Radio and TV talk shows have been organized at all levels of health care delivery. The RHNP has trained 1,000 change agents. Health walks have been organized with by increasing frequency by the general public, corporate bodies, civil service organizations and religious organizations for their general health benefits and to draw attention to various social issues (GNA, 2007, 2009b). Some of the health walks have been accompanied by free HIV/AIDS testing and counselling, blood pressure and weight checks and eye care. Despite these efforts, general awareness of NCDs, their causes, effect, prevention and treatment remains low(Clegg-Lamptey and Hodasi, 2000; Spencer et al., 2005), even among medical professionals (Adanu, 2002). The situation is compounded by the paucity of educational materials on NCDs in health facilities.

The media visibility of health screening programmes has also been increasing. Screening programmes for weight, height, blood pressure, breast and cervical cancers have generally been led by NGOs although female parliamentarians have also contributed to raising awareness. The increased availability of equipment (e.g. ultrasound, weighing scales, mammography) and laboratory tests (e.g. pap smear, prostate specific antigen) in both the public and private sector favours screening programmes. An aide memoire signed between MOH and development partners in November 2007 called for the introduction of structured programme of health screening as a priority in 2008 (MOH, 2007). Accordingly, the government of Ghana, in its 2008 budget, planned to promote greater awareness of early detection of breast and prostate cancer; and introduce a programme for breast and prostate cancer screening. Further, the government decided to subsidize mammograms done in private and public hospitals for all Ghanaian women from the age of 40 years and above and for prostate cancer screening for men of 50 years and above who are registered under the NHIS (Republic of Ghana, 2008). This plan is yet to be implemented due to funding constraints.

The chronic shortage of equipment, logistics and drugs in the 1980s before the introduction of the 'cash and carry' user fee scheme in the early 1990s is no longer an issue. Following some GHS quality assurance training programmes, many regional and district hospitals now use sphygmomanometers, weighing scales and height measures in open spaces in outpatient departments. Despite this favourable development, missed opportunities exist. It is not uncommon for an obese patient with malaria or a smoker with diarrhoea to receive treatment for the acute illness without any counselling or care of their relevant NCD risk factors. This is even more pertinent as clinicians are effective in achieving risk factor reduction (Gorin and Heck, 2004).

A Newborn Screening for Sickle Cell Disease (NSSCD) project was started in Kumasi and Tikrom in the Ashanti Region in April 2003 with funding from the National Institute of Health (Ohene-Frimpong et al., 2008). The project officially ended in March 2008 and has contributed to early detection of SCD and improved clinical outcomes. Based on the success of the project, the Ghana Health Service, in collaboration with the Sickle Cell Foundation of Ghana, has started to scale up the neonatal screening to other parts of the Ashanti Region and then to the rest of the country.

With regard to clinical management, the challenges include the general absence of national treatment guidelines, multiplicity of treatment regimens, high cost of treatment, low compliance with treatment, high defaulter rate, recourse to unlicensed herbal products and shortage of specialist care. Several studies have shown that treatment and control of hypertension is low (Agyemang et al., 2006; Amoah, 2003). The implementation of a National Health Insurance Scheme (NHIS) in Ghana in March 2005 has provided substantial financial relief for the growing list of registered participants. The benefit package includes common medications for outpatient and inpatient care, ultrasound and laboratory investigations, physiotherapy and some surgical operations (GHS, 2004). However, it excludes some cardiac investigations (e.g. echocardiography, angiography), some anti-hypertensive drugs (e.g. candesartan, ramipril), therapy for cancers other than for breast and cervical cancers, and prosthetic devices (NHIA, 2007).

For tertiary prevention, Limb Fitting Centres, and occupational and physiotherapy centres in the few public facilities where they are available are chronically under-funded and so lack modern equipment. However, since 1998, the three newer regional hospitals in the Central, Brong-Ahafo and Volta regions as well as the teaching hospitals have modern physiotherapy equipment. Palliative care is sub-optimal, with few trained physicians. There appears to be a general reluctance to use morphine and other narcotics for pain relief, probably due to fear of addiction.

There are several other cross-cutting challenges. Recent national assessments of care services in health facilities in Ghana have excluded NCDs (GSS et al., 2003; MOH, 2007b). The last review of capacity for NCD care was undertaken in five regional hospitals for diabetes in 1995 (Amoah et al., 1998). The NCDCP has not formally been evaluated since it was established in 1992. In comparison, the National Tuberculosis Programme, which was established in 1994, has been evaluated at least five times. The RHNP was the focus of in-depth review during the health sector review of 2007 (MOH, 2008). Funding for NCDs has been woefully inadequate though that for the RHNP is relatively good. Many development partners are not interested in NCDs, preferring to support infectious diseases and programmes with quicker impact.

What Ghana needs to do

Ghana has to implement the recommendations of the sixtieth WHA resolution of 2007 (WHO, 2007):

1. Strengthen national and local political will to prevent and control NCDs.
2. Establish and strengthen a national multisectoral coordinating mechanism for prevention and control of NCDs.
3. Finalize and implement a national multisectoral evidence-based action plan for prevention and control of NCDs that sets out priorities, a time frame and performance indicators.
4. Increase resources for programmes for the prevention and control of NCDs.
5. Implement existing global initiatives and the Framework Convention on Tobacco Control.
6. Strengthen the capacity of health systems for prevention, to integrate prevention and control of NCDs into primary health-care programmes.
7. Strengthen monitoring and evaluation systems, including country-level epidemiological surveillance mechanisms.
8. Strengthen the role of governmental regulatory functions in combating NCDs.
9. Increase access to appropriate health care including affordable, high-quality medicines.
10. Implement public health interventions to reduce the incidence of obesity in children and adults.

Opportunities

While the challenges may seem daunting, there are a number of opportunities that the health sector could exploit. The government has determined to process nine health-related bills including the tobacco bill for passage into law. There is also public support for a ban on public smoking – a recent survey showed that 80 percent of workers in smoking and non-smoking establishments were in favour of smoke-free laws (GNA, 2009c). Health promotion campaigns should take advantage of the changing cultural perceptions of Ghanaian women on preferred body size and shape. Overweight Ghanaian women are interested and willing to reduce their body size for health and cosmetic reasons (Duda et al., 2006; Mallet, 2004).

Increased provides the opportunity for facilities to expand their services. For example, the uptake of clients screened for cervical cancer using visual inspection with acetic acid (VIA) at the Ridge Hospital in Accra increased five-fold from 161 to 818 within the second quarter of 2007 and 2008 following an educational programme on VIA on one television network (Ridge Hospital Family Planning Centre, 2009). Funding from better-resourced 'vertical' programmes should be managed horizontally towards health system strengthening (e.g. for health promotion, training and surveillance) for the benefit of less-endowed programmes.

The recently introduced District Health Information Management System (DHIMS) as an integral tool to capture preventive and clinical service output in private and public health facilities in Ghana should provide more timely and accurate NCD-related data at the district and regional levels (MOH, 2009). The recent introduction of selected NCDs into the national integrated disease surveillance and response (IDSR) system, although not fully implemented, could help to improve surveillance on NCDs and garner health worker interest in NCDs. Periodic national surveys such as the GDHS and the Multiple Indicator Cluster Survey generate accurate data on nutritional status and tobacco that are useful for monitoring risk factor trends in adults and in children.

There are other opportunities to improve clinical care. The recently developed clinical protocols for diabetes by the International Diabetes Federation African Region, cardiovascular risk assessment guidelines and a Package of Essential NCD (WHO-PEN) interventions for the prevention and control of four major NCDs at the primary care level could be adapted for national use (IDF, 2006; WHO, 2007). Unlike the medical associations of UK and US, the Ghana Medical Association has not recently developed any monographs or scientific papers on NCDs although it has the capacity to do so (BMA, 2008; Kushner, 2003). Since 2007, the new requirement by the Ghana Medical and Dental Council for doctors and dental officers to accumulate 20 credit points for re-licensure each year has enabled a large number of doctors to receive training updates in some NCDs. Where specialists are not available, outreach specialist sessions could improve the clinical management of NCDs at the periphery.

Besides expanding the coverage and benefit package of the NHIS, medicinal plant research could potentially reduce the cost of medicines (Nyarko et al., 2004; Quaye et al., 2004). More NCD-related research is needed. Thus, the recent formation of the research consortium – UK Africa Academic Partnership on Chronic Disease (www.appcafrica.org) -- is commendable.

In the health sector performance review 2008, the independent team concluded that the running of parallel NCD programmes—the RHNP by the MOH and the NCDCP by the GHS— is inefficient (MOH, 2009). There is scope for the two programmes to be integrated for more effective use of resources. A proposed restructuring of disease control programmes within the Ghana Health Service to elevate the status of the NCDCP and appoint Focal Persons to the NCDCP should serve to attract more funding for more effective programme management.

Conclusions

Non-communicable diseases have increased substantially in Ghana and they are likely to continue to do so. Ghana has had a chequered history of several laudable policy initiatives which have not been fully followed through for implementation and evaluation. Several opportunities exist to improve the policy and programmatic response to NCDs using a multisectoral and integrated approach.

References

Adanu R.M. (200).Cervical cancer knowledge and screening in Accra, Ghana. *J Womens Health Gend Based Med*.**11**:487-488.

African Hebrew Development Agency. Regenerative Health & Nutrition Programme Annual Report 2007; March 2008.

Agyemang C. (2006).Rural and urban differences in blood pressure and hypertension in Ghana, *West Africa. Public Health*;**120**(6):525-533.

Agyemang, C., Bruijnzeels ,M.A., Owusu-Dabo, E.(2006). Factors associated with hypertension awareness, treatment, and control in Ghana, West Africa. *Journal of Human Hypertension.* **20**:67-71.

Amoah, A.G.B.(2003) Hypertension in Ghana: A cross-sectional community prevalence study in Greater Accra. *Ethn Dis* . **13**:310-315.

Amoah A.G., Owusu, S.K., Saunders. J.T., Fang, W.L., Asare, H.A., Pastors, J.G., et al. (1998). Facilities and resources for diabetes care at regional health facilities in southern Ghana. *Diabetes Res Clin Pract.* **42**:123-130.

Amoah, A.G., Owusu, S.K., Acheampong, J.W., Agyenim-Boateng, K., Asare, H.R, Owusu, A.A. et al. (2000). A national diabetes care and education programme: the Ghana model. *Diabetes Res Clin Pract* **49**:149-157.

Amoah, A.G., Owusu .S.K., Adjei S. (2002).Diabetes in Ghana: a community based prevalence study in Greater Accra. *Diabetes Research and Clinical Practice. 56:197-205.*

Biritwum, R., Gyapong,J., Mensah, G. (2005).The epidemiology of obesity in Ghana. *Ghana Med J.* **39**:82-85.

Bosu, W.K. (2008).Position Paper on the Prevention and Control of National Non-Communicable Diseases in Ghana Accra: GHS Ghana.

British Medical Association. Alcohol misuse: tackling the UK epidemic; February 2008.

Cappuccio, F.P., Micah, F.B., Emmett, L, Kerry, S.M., Antwi, S., Martin-Peprah. R, et al. (2004). Prevalence, detection, management, and control of hypertension in Ashanti, *West Africa. Hyperten*s;**43**:1017-1022.

Clegg-Lamptey, J.N.A., Hodasi, W.M. (2000).A study of breast cancer in Korle-bu Teaching Hospital: Assessing the impact of health education. *Ghana Med J.***41**:72-77.

Colbourne, M.J., Edington, G.M., Hughes, M.H., Ward-Brew, A. (1950). A medical survey in a gold coast village. *Trans R Soc Trop Med Hyg.* **44**:271-290.

Dodu, S.R.A.(1950).The incidence of diabetes mellitus in Accra (Ghana): A study of 4000 patients. *West Afr Med J*:129-134.

Duda, R.B., Jumah .N.A., Hill, A,G., Seffah. J., Biritwum R. (2006). Interest in healthy living outweighs presumed cultural norms for obesity for Ghanaian women. Health and Quality of Life Outcomes;**4**.

Duda, R.B., Kim. M.P., Darko, R., Adanu., R.M., Seffah, J., Anarfi, J.K,.et al. (2007). Results of the Women's Health Study of Accra: assessment of blood pressure in urban women. *Int J Cardiol* **117**:115-122.

Ghana Health Service. (2004). National Health Insurance: a handbook for service providers. Accra; August 2004.

Ghana News Agency. (2007). Ghanaians walk for health. 6 October 2007 [cited 7 August 2009]; Available from: http://www.ghanaweb.com/GhanaHomePage/NewsArchive/artikel.php?ID=131948

Ghana News Agency. (2009a) Tobacco bill to go before cabinet soon. General News 3 July 2009 Available from: http://www.ghanaweb.com/GhanaHomePage/NewsArchive/artikel.php?ID=164763. [cited 7 August 2009]

Ghana News Agency. (2009b) Madina Muslim community to undertake health walk. 30 April 2009 [cited 7 August 2009]; Available from: http://www.ghanaweb.com/GhanaHomePage/NewsArchive/artikel.php?ID=161379

Ghana News Agency. (2009c). Anti-tobacco law gains support. 29 May 2009 [cited 7 August 2009]; Available from: http://www.ghanaweb.com/GhanaHomePage/NewsArchive/artikel.php?ID=162885

Ghana Statistical Service, Health Research Unit, ORC Macro. Ghana Service Provision Assessment (2002). Calverton, Maryland: GSS and ORC Macro; August 2003.

Ghana Statistical Service, (2004).Macro International Inc., Noguchi Memorial Institute for Medical Research. Ghana Demographic and Health Survey 2003. Claverton, Maryland: GSS and MI; 2004.

Ghana Statistical Service (GSS), Ghana Health Service (GHS), ICF Macro. Ghana Demographic and Health Survey (2008). Accra, Ghana: GSS, GHS and ICF Macro; 2009.

Gorin, S.S., Heck, J.E.(2004). Meta-analysis of the efficacy of tobacco counseling by health care providers. *Cancer Epidemiol Biomarkers Prev***13**:2012-2022.

Haddock, D.R.W. (1970). Cerebrovascular accidents in Ghana. *Trans R Soc Trop Med Hyg* . **64**:300-310.

Hall, J.N., Moore, S., Harper, S.B., Lynch, J.W. (2009). Global variability in fruit and vegetable consumption. *Am J Prev Med* .**36**:402-409.

Health Interventions Group. (2001).Priority Health Interventions in Ghana. Accra: GHS;

Hill, A.G., Darko, R., Seffah, J., Adanu, R.M.K., Anarfi, J.K., Duda, R.B. (2007). Health of urban ,Ghanaian women as identified by the Women's Health Study of *Accra. Int J Gyn Obstet.* **99**:150-156.

Ikeme, A.C., Pole D.J., Pobee, J.O., Larbi, E., Blankson., J., Williams, H. (1978). Cardiovascular status and blood pressure in a population sample in Ghana--the Mamprobi survey. *Trop Geogr Med* . **30**:313-329.

International Diabetes Federation African Region. (July 2006.)Diabetes education training manual for Sub-Saharan Africa: IDF, WDF.

Kushner, R.F. (2003). Roadmaps for Clinical Practice: Case Studies in Disease Prevention and Health Promotion—Assessment and Management of Adult Obesity: A Primer for Physicians. Chicago, Illinois: *American Medical Association*;

Mallet. B. (2004). Do Ghanaian ladies care about their body sizes? A case study of perceptions about body size and anthropometry of University of Ghana female students. Abstract no. Fourth Annual Research Meeting and 25th Anniversary celebrations, 22-24 Nov, 2004. Accra: Noguchi Memorial Institute for Medical Research, University of Ghana.

Martorell, R., Khan, K.L, Hughes, M.L, Grummer-Strawn, LM. (2000)Obesity in women from developing countries. *Eur J Clin Nutr.* **54**:247-252.

Ministry of Health Ghana. (1994). Policies and priorities for the health sector 1994-1995. Accra: MOH.;

Ministry of Health Ghana. (1995a) Medium term health strategy: towards Vision 2020. Accra: MOH; September 1995.

Ministry of Health Ghana. (1995b) Report of the seminar on non-communicable diseases at the Clinical Lecture Theatre, Dept of Medicine, Korle Bu, 8-9 June 1995. Accra: MOH; 1995.

Ministry of Health Ghana. Health(1996). sector 5 Year Programme of Work. Accra: MOH; August.

Ministry of Health Ghana. (1998).Strategy Paper on Non–communicable Diseases Control Programme. Accra: MOH; March .

Ministry of Health Ghana. (2001). The Health of the Nation: reflections on the first five year health sector programme of work 1997-2001. Accra: MOH; August

Ministry of Health Ghana. (2002).Non–communicable Diseases Control Programme: draft policy. Accra: MOH; March.

Ministry of Health Ghana. (2007a) National health policy: creating wealth through health. Accra: MOH; September .

Ministry of Health Ghana. (2007b)Joint Ministry of Health-Development Partners Health Summit, GIMPA: Aide memoir. Accra: MOH; 19-23 Nov.

Ministry of Health Ghana. (2007c) Service Availability Mapping (SAM). Accra: MOH, WHO, DFID; April ..

Ministry of Health Ghana. (2008a) Regenerative Health & Nutrition Strategic Plan 2007- 2011. Accra: MOH.

Ministry of Health Ghana. (2008b) The Ghana Health Sector 5 Year Programme of Work 2007-20011: Creating Wealth through Health. Accra: MOH; February

Ministry of Health Ghana. (2008c) Independent Review Health Sector Programme Of Work 2007. Accra: MOH; April .

Ministry of Health Ghana. (2009).Independent Review of Ghana Health Sector Programme of Work 2008: pulling together, achieving more. Accra: MOH; May

National Health Insurance Authority. National Health Insurance Scheme Medicines List, effective January 2008. Accra: NHIA; 2007.

Non-communicable Disease Control Programme. Annual Report (2001). Accra: Ghana Health Service; 2002.

Non-communicable Disease Control Programme. Report on a 2-Day Workshop on Integrated Control and Prevention of Non Communicable Diseases and Injuries 8-9 June 2005. Accra: GHS; July 2005.

Nyame, P.K., Bonsu-Bruce, N., Amoah, A.G., Adjei, S., Nyarko, E., Amuah, E.A. et al. (1994) Current trends in the incidence of cerebrovascular accidents in Accra. *West Afr J Med* 1994;**13**:183-186.

Nyarko, A., Ofori-Adjei, D., Sittie, A.A., Bastow, K.N., Lee, K.H.(20040. Anti-tumour effects of selected Ghanaian medicinal plants. Fourth Annual Research Meeting and 25th Anniversary celebrations, 22-24 Nov, 2004. Accra: Noguchi Memorial Institute for Medical Research, University of Ghana.

Ohene-Frempong, K., Oduro, J., Tetteh, H., Nkrumah, F. (2008).Screening newborns for sickle cell disease in Ghana. *Pediatrics* . **121**(Suppl 2):120-121.

Owiredu, W.K.B.A., Adamu, M.S., Amidu, N., Woode, E., Bam, V., Plange-Rhule ,J., et al. (2008). Obesity and Cardiovascular Risk Factors in a Pentecostal Population in Kumasi-*Ghana. J Med Sci*. **8**:682-690.

Pobee, J.O. 91993). Community-based high blood pressure programs in sub-Saharan Africa. *Ethn Dis* **3 Suppl**:S38-45.

Pobee, J.O.M.(2006). The Heart of the Matter: Community profile of cardiovascular diseases of a sub-Saharan African country.The Ghanaian Paradigm.The Mamprobi Cardiovascular Health Project 1975-1983. Accra: University of Ghana..

Quaye, O., Nyarko ,A. Addy, M.E., Okine, L.KN. (2004) Acute and subchronic toxicity studies of an anti-asthmatic and anti-inflammatory plant medicine AN2000. Fourth Annual Research Meeting and 25th Anniversary celebrations, 22-24 Nov, 2004. Accra: Noguchi Memorial Institute for Medical Research, University of Ghana; 2004.

Republic of Ghana. (2008).The Budget Statement and Economic Policy of the Government of Ghana for the 2008 Financial Year. Accra: MOFEP.

Ridge Hospital Family Planning Centre.(2009). Annual Report 2008 . Accra: GHS; .

Sackey, S.O.(1993). Draft programme document: non-communicable diseases control programme. Accra: MOH Ghana.

Spencer, .J, Phillips, E.., Ogedegbe, G. (2005). Knowledge attitudes, beliefs, and blood pressure control in a community-based sample in Ghana. *Ethnicity and Disease* **15**:748-752.

West Africa Health Organization. (2006).Double burden of malnutrition in West Africa. 10th ECOWAS Nutrition Forum. Mindelo: ECOWAS; 22 September 2006.

World Health Organization. (2007a) Prevention and control of noncommunicable diseases: implementation of the global strategy. WHA60.23, 23 May 2007. Geneva: WHO.

World Health Organization. (2007b) Prevention of cardiovascular disease : pocket guidelines for assessment and management of cardiovascular risk : (WHO/ISH cardiovascular risk prediction charts for the African Region. Geneva: WHO.

World Health Organization. (2008a) 2008-2013 action plan for the global strategy for the prevention and control of noncommunicable diseases : prevent and control cardiovascular diseases, cancers, chronic respiratory diseases and diabetes. Geneva: WHO.

WHO. (2008b) Ouagadougou Declaration on Primary Health Care and Health Systems in Africa: achieving better health for Africa in the new millennium. Ouagadougou.

WHO Regional Office for Africa. (2000). Noncommunicable diseases: A strategy for the African Region. AFR/RC50/10. Harare: WHO AFRO.

WHO Regional Office for Africa. Cardiovascular diseases in the African Region: current situation and perspectives. AFR/RC55/12, Maputo, 17 June 2005. Brazzaville: WHO AFRO..

WHO Regional Office for Africa. (2007a) Diabetes prevention and control: A strategy for the WHO African Region. AFR/RC57/7. Brazzaville: WHO AFRO.

WHO Regional Office for Africa. (2007b) Food safety and health: A strategy for the WHO African Region. AFR/RC57/4, 25 June 2007. Brazzaville: WHO AFRO;

WHO Regional Office for Africa. (2007c). Harmful use of alcohol in the WHO African Region: situation analysis and perspectives. AFR/RC57/14. Brazzaville: WHO AFRO.

WHO Regional Office for Africa. (2008a) Cancer prevention and control: A strategy for the WHO African Region. AFR/RC58/4, Yaounde, 24 June 2008. Brazzaville: WHO AFRO.

WHO Regional Office for Africa. (2008b) Implementation of the Framework Convention on Tobacco Control in the African Region: current status and the way forward. AFR/RC55/13, Maputo, 17 June 2005. Brazzaville: WHO AFRO..

Table 9.1: Recent WHO Resolutions on Non-Communicable Diseases and Health Promotion

Year	Strategy or initiative	Code	Thematic Area
May 1998	WHA request for a global strategy for NCD prevention and control	WHA51.18	NCDs
May 2000	Reaffirmation of global strategy for prevention and control of NCDs	WHA53.17	NCDs
May 2001	Transparency in tobacco control process	WHA54.18	Tobacco
May 2002	Development of a Global Strategy on Diet, Physical Activity and Health (DPAS)	WHA53.23	DPAS
May 2003	Adoption of WHO Framework Convention on Tobacco Control (FCTC)	WHA56.1	Tobacco
May 2004	Endorsement of DPAS	WHA57.17	DPAS
May 2004	Health promotion and healthy lifestyles	WHA57.16	Health promotion
May 2005	Cancer prevention and control	WHA58.22	Cancers
May 2005	Public health problems caused by harmful use of alcohol	WHA58.26	Alcohol
May 2006	Sickle-cell anaemia	WHA59.20	Sickle cell disease
May 2007	Prevention and control of NCDs: implementation of the global strategy. Call to prepare an action plan	WHA60.23	NCDs
May 2008	Endorsement of a six-year Global Action Plan 2008-2013	WHA61.14	NCDs
2008	MPOWER policies on tobacco control	-	Tobacco

Index

I

infectious diseases xi, 1, 2, 3, 4, 29, 129, 130, 147

K

Kintampo 6, 45, 46, 47, 74, 89, 108

Komfo Anokye Teaching Hospital xiii, 31, 33, 37, 43, 49, 59, 96, 106

Korle-Bu Teaching Hospital xiii, 28, 30, 31, 33, 37, 43, 51, 59, 68, 89, 134, 137, 139

Kumasi xi, 1, 6, 33, 34, 35, 37, 40, 44, 49, 51, 52, 53, 59, 67, 68, 73, 76, 77, 78, 92, 98, 99, 100, 104, 106, 113, 138, 141, 146, 154

L

lifestyle(s) viii, 2, 3, 4, 7, 22, 23, 24, 29, 41, 48, 74, 75, 76, 78, 109, 110, 115, 116, 122, 124, 125, 131, 142, 143, 145, 156

M

mental disorders vii, xiii, 2, 89, 91, 92, 94, 95, 96, 98, 99, 101, 102, 103, 106

mental health vii, xi, 1, 3, 6, 8, 10, 88, 89, 90, 96, 97, 98, 99, 101, 102, 103, 104, 105, 107

mental health bill 88

mental illness xi, xii, 1, 88, 91, 92, 93, 94, 95, 97, 98, 99, 100, 101, 102, 103, 106, 107

Millennium Development Goals (MDGs) xiii, 8

Ministry of Health xiii, 11, 26, 84, 138, 139, 153, 154

morbidity viii, x, 2, 4, 8, 9, 13, 29, 31, 41, 48, 53, 56, 72, 91, 93, 106, 116, 132, 138, 139

mortality viii, x, 1, 2, 4, 8, 9, 24, 26, 28, 29, 30, 31, 34, 39, 40, 48, 53, 56, 60, 61, 68, 115, 116, 122, 132, 133, 135, 136

multi-morbid conditions 4

N

neurodegenerative diseases ix, 3

Nkoranza 6, 45, 46, 47

O

obesity viii, x, 5, 9, 10, 11, 13, 31, 40, 51, 52, 71, 110, 111, 112, 116, 119, 120, 121, 122, 124, 125, 126, 127, 130, 133, 134, 135, 138, 141, 148, 151

over-nutrition 4, 5

overweight viii, 5, 110, 112, 127, 145

P

physical activity x, 14, 17, 21, 22, 24, 110, 115, 119, 121, 125, 127, 136, 143

physical inactivity viii, 13, 109, 116, 124, 125

poverty 2, 3, 4, 5, 8, 46, 95, 124, 127, 129, 130, 131

Prevention, primary 22, 23, 26, 28, 54, 84, 121, 144

Prevention, secondary 145

Prevention, tertiary 38, 145, 147

psychosis 2, 88, 89, 92, 93, 95, 96, 98, 99, 101, 103, 105

psychotic illness 92, 93, 99

R

Religion 64, 68

S

schizophrenia 2, 90, 92, 93, 99, 107

sickle-cell disease 1, 6, 139

smoking 3, 51, 71, 110, 112, 113, 116, 121, 124, 125, 127, 130, 131, 140, 141, 144, 148

social support 6, 42, 46, 50, 129

sorcery 45

stigma 35, 37, 47, 54, 62, 100, 102, 134

stigmatization 33, 35, 62

stroke iv, vii, viii, xii, 1, 5, 13, 24, 26, 27, 29, 30, 31, 32, 33, 34, 35, 36, 37, 38, 39, 40, 41, 54, 109, 128, 129, 135

sub-Saharan Africa vii, 11, 14, 23, 25, 27, 29, 30, 40, 49, 54, 72, 74, 76, 80, 81, 112, 122, 124, 132, 136, 154

T

Tema 6, 43, 45, 68

traditional healer 99

traditional healing 6, 100, 107

traditional medicine 6, 131

Transition

demographic 2, 3

epidemiological 2, 4, 11, 129, 135, 136

health 2, 3

nutrition 2, 4, 9, 11, 122

U

under-nutrition 4, 5, 130, 143

urbanization viii, 3, 4, 28, 29, 36, 38, 86, 109, 126, 131

V

vegetable consumption 138, 141, 152

W

wheeze 74, 75, 77, 80, 84, 86
wheezing 70, 71, 74
witchcraft 45, 93, 94, 128, 132
World Health Organization (WHO 12, 29, 70, 137